T0191940

Emergency Department Management of Obstetric Complications

Joelle Borhart

Editor

Emergency Department Management of Obstetric Complications

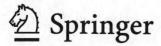 Springer

Editor
Joelle Borhart
MedStar Georgetown University Hospital and
MedStar Washington Hospital Center
Georgetown University School of Medicine
Washington, DC
USA

ISBN 978-3-319-85388-8   ISBN 978-3-319-54410-6   (eBook)
DOI 10.1007/978-3-319-54410-6

Printed on acid-free paper

This Springer imprint is published by Springer Nature
The registered company is Springer International Publishing AG
The registered company address is: Gewerbestrasse 11, 6330 Cham, Switzerland

Preface

Obstetrical emergencies can be among the most stressful events an emergency physician will face in their entire career. Late pregnancy bleeding or a precipitous emergency department (ED) delivery can provoke anxiety in even the most seasoned emergency physician. Trauma and cardiovascular emergencies in pregnant patients can result in catastrophic outcomes for both mother and baby. When it comes to pregnant patients, even seemingly minor presentations such as trip and fall can become an area of treachery.

The goal of this book is to provide an evidence-based, practical approach to the wide spectrum of obstetric complications an emergency physician must be prepared to manage throughout all trimesters of pregnancy as well as postpartum. The approach to the pregnant patient with trauma, with non-pregnancy-related abdominal pain, or in cardiac arrest is discussed. Updates in the classification and management of the hypertensive disorders of pregnancy are presented. Recent controversies surrounding the use of antiemetics for first-trimester nausea and vomiting and the use of a beta-hCG discriminatory zone for the evaluation of pregnancy of unknown location are also addressed.

This book is written for emergency clinicians in all practice settings. Obstetrical support services vary widely between different facilities, and emergency physicians must be prepared to initially manage any pregnant patient that comes through the door. It is my hope that this book provides useful information for daily practice as well as preparation for rarely encountered and potentially life-threatening events.

The departmental leadership of the MedStar Georgetown University and MedStar Washington Hospital Center Emergency Departments was incredibly supportive of this project, and I am grateful for their assistance. I would like to thank the Emergency Medicine Residency Program faculty and residents for their contributions, encouragement, and friendship. The authors of all the chapters deserve recognition for their outstanding contributions to this text. My son Sean, born during the production of this book, has been a source of inspiration, joy, and reminder of what is most important in life. Finally, I must thank my husband, Steve—you took on far more than your share of household duties and childcare to allow me the time to complete this project. Without your support, this book would not have been possible.

Emergency physicians are in a unique position to have a potentially tremendous impact on the life of a pregnant patient and her unborn child. I hope that this book equips you with the tools to provide the best possible care for your obstetric patients in the ED each and every day.

Washington, DC   Joelle Borhart, M.D., F.A.C.E.P., F.A.A.E.M.

Contents

List of Contributors

Elaine Bromberek, M.D. Department of Emergency Medicine, MedStar Georgetown University and MedStar Washington Hospital Center, Washington, DC, USA

Christina Bird, D.O. Department of Emergency Medicine, UT Health Science Center, San Antonio, TX, USA

Joelle Borhart, M.D. Department of Emergency Medicine, MedStar Georgetown University Hospital and MedStar Washington Hospital Center, Washington, DC, USA

Lisel Curtis, M.D Department of Emergency Medicine, MedStar Georgetown University Hospital, Washington, DC, USA

Lindsey DeGeorge, M.D. Department of Emergency Medicine, MedStar Washington Hospital Center, Washington, DC, USA

Edward Descallar, M.D. Department of Emergency Medicine, MedStar Georgetown University Hospital and MedStar Washington Hospital Center, Washington, DC, USA

Kayla Dewey, M.D. Department of Emergency Medicine, MedStar Washington Hospital Center and MedStar Georgetown University, Washington, DC, USA

Maria Dynin, M.D. Department of Emergency Medicine, MedStar Georgetown University Hospital, Washington, DC, USA

Julie Gorchynski, M.D. Department of Emergency Medicine, UT Health Science Center, San Antonio, TX, USA

Linda Hatch, M.D. Department of Emergency Medicine, UT Health Science Center, San Antonio, TX, USA

Diana Ladkany, B.S., M.D. Department of Emergency Medicine, MedStar Washington Hospital Center and MedStar Georgetown University, Washington, DC, USA

David R. Lane, M.D. Department of Emergency Medicine, MedStar Southern Maryland Hospital Center, Clinton, MD, USA

Kerri Layman, B.S.F.S., M.D., R.D.M.S Department of Emergency Medicine, MedStar Georgetown University Hospital and MedStar Washington Hospital Center, Washington, DC, USA

Marcos Mavromaras, M.D. Department of Emergency Medicine, UT Health Science Center, San Antonio, TX, USA

Jessica Palmer, M.D. Department of Emergency Medicine, MedStar Southern Maryland Hospital, Clinton, MD, USA

Erica Peethumnongsin, M.D. Division of Emergency Medicine, Department of Surgery, Duke University Hospital, Durham, NC, USA

Carolyn Phillips, M.D., R.D.M.S. Department of Emergency Medicine, MedStar Washington Hospital Center and MedStar Georgetown University, Washington, DC, USA

Elizabeth Pontius, M.D., R.D.M.S. Department of Emergency Medicine, MedStar Washington Hospital Center, Washington, DC, USA

Brian Sharp, M.D., F.A.C.E.P. BerbeeWalsh Department of Emergency Medicine, University of Wisconsin, Madison, WI, USA

Kristen Sharp, M.D. Department of Obstetrics and Gynecology, University of Wisconsin, Madison, WI, USA

Mallory Shasteen, M.D. Department of Emergency Medicine, Greenville Hospital System, Greenville, SC, USA

Lili Sheibani, M.D. Division of Maternal-Fetal Medicine, Department of Obstetrics and Gynecology, Keck School of Medicine, USC, Los Angeles, CA, USA

Whitney Sherman, M.D. Department of Emergency Medicine, MedStar Georgetown University Hospital and MedStar Washington Hospital Center, Washington, DC, USA

Janet Smereck, M.D. Department of Emergency Medicine, MedStar Georgetown University Hospital, Washington, DC, USA

Nick Tsipis, M.D. Department of Emergency Medicine, MedStar Georgetown University Hospital and MedStar Washington Hospital Center, Washington, DC, USA

Kathryn Voss, M.D. Department of Emergency Medicine, MedStar Washington Hospital Center and MedStar Georgetown University, Washington, DC, USA

Marianne Wallis, M.D. Department of Emergency Medicine, MedStar Georgetown University Hospital and MedStar Washington Hospital Center, Washington, DC, USA

Eric Wei, M.D., M.B.A. Department of Emergency Medicine, LAC+USC Medical Center, Los Angeles, CA, USA

Lauren Wiesner, M.D. Department of Emergency Medicine, MedStar Washington Hospital Center, Washington, DC, USA

Cory Wittrock, M.D. Department of Emergency Medicine, MedStar Georgetown University Hospital, Washington, DC, USA

Chapter 1
Early Pregnancy Complications

Kayla Dewey, Kathryn Voss, and Carolyn Phillips

Introduction

Pregnant patients often present to the emergency department (ED) with chief complaints of abdominal pain and/or vaginal bleeding in the first trimester. Women presenting to the ED in early pregnancy may not be aware of their pregnancy status; it is critical that emergency clinicians test for pregnancy in any woman of childbearing age with abdominal pain or vaginal bleeding. Helpful historical clues include date of last menstrual period (LMP) and, for patients who are aware they are pregnant, whether or not they have had an ultrasound with this pregnancy.

Complications such as pain and bleeding in early pregnancy are common. Indeed, one fourth of women will have vaginal bleeding or spotting in the first few weeks of pregnancy, and one half of those patients will miscarry [1]. Ultimately these patients will receive a diagnosis of threatened miscarriage, miscarriage, pregnancy of unknown location, ectopic pregnancy, or, rarely, heterotopic pregnancy. Some complications such as ectopic pregnancy may be life threatening; others are emotionally devastating and may impact future fertility. Emergency physicians must be prepared to evaluate and manage the various complications of early pregnancy.

K. Dewey, M.D. (✉) • K. Voss, M.D. • C. Phillips, M.D., R.D.M.S.
Department of Emergency Medicine, MedStar Washington Hospital Center and MedStar Georgetown University, 110 Irving St. NW, Washington, DC 20010, USA
e-mail: kayla.dewey@gmail.com; voss.kathryn@gmail.com; carolynaphillips@gmail.com

© Springer International Publishing AG 2017
J. Borhart (ed.), *Emergency Department Management of Obstetric Complications*,
DOI 10.1007/978-3-319-54410-6_1

Ectopic Pregnancy

The most concerning diagnosis for the first trimester pregnant patient is ectopic pregnancy, defined as any pregnancy outside the uterus. It remains the highest cause of mortality for pregnant women in the first trimester in the United States [2]. Ectopic pregnancy is estimated to occur in 2% of all pregnancies; however, the incidence of ectopic pregnancy among ED patients who present with abdominal pain and/or vaginal bleeding in the first trimester is as high as 13–16% [2, 3]. The incidence of ectopic pregnancies has been increasing, thought to reflect increases in rates of pelvic inflammatory disease and the use of assisted reproductive technologies (ART). It is imperative that clinicians are knowledgeable about the diagnosis, management, and appropriate disposition for these high-risk patients.

While ectopic pregnancy is defined as a pregnancy in any location that is outside the uterus, the majority occur within the fallopian tube, with 93–97% implanting in the distal portion of the tube [2]. Rarely, pregnancy can occur within the ovary, the abdominal cavity, the cervix, or adjacent to Cesarean scar tissue. The final common pathway for ectopic pregnancies is a delay or prevention of passage of an embryo through the fallopian tube and into the uterine cavity. Proposed mechanisms include anatomic obstruction, abnormalities of ciliary function or other motility mechanisms, abnormal embryo formation, and chemotactic factors that favor tubal implantation [4]. For a tubal ectopic pregnancy, the growth of the embryo is limited by the vascular supply and anatomic size of the fallopian tube; β-hCG levels will plateau or fall when embryonic development cannot continue normally. Vaginal bleeding may be the result of sloughing of the endometrium, from invasion of the embryo into the mucosa of the tube itself or from rupture causing hemoperitoneum [2].

Half of all ectopic pregnancies occur in patients without any known risk factors. Traditionally, prior ectopic pregnancy, prior tubal surgery or other tubal pathology, history of pelvic inflammatory disease, maternal smoking, and age over 35 were all associated with increased risk [5, 6]. More recently, increased use of ART has become an independent risk factor. The use of intrauterine devices (IUD) has not been shown to contribute to overall risk, but when pregnancy does occur in a patient with an IUD, it is more likely to be ectopic than intrauterine [4].

Clinical presentations of ectopic pregnancy can vary widely. Most commonly, patients complain of abdominal pain and vaginal bleeding. Many are unaware they are pregnant prior to ED presentation, and these patients may report a missed, delayed, or abnormal menstrual cycle. Clinical signs of ectopic pregnancy will vary based on gestational age, location, and whether or not the ectopic has ruptured. Ruptured ectopic pregnancies often present acutely with evidence of severe abdominal tenderness and adnexal mass on physical exam and can progress to hypovolemic shock. History of focal pain that was severe but progressed to generalized pain and symptoms of peritoneal irritation are also consistent with a ruptured ectopic. However, the majority of patients present prior to rupture and ectopic pregnancy can go undiagnosed on the first ED visit.

Fig. 1.1 Transabdominal ultrasound in a patient with a ruptured ectopic pregnancy showing free fluid and echogenic fluid from the hemorrhage

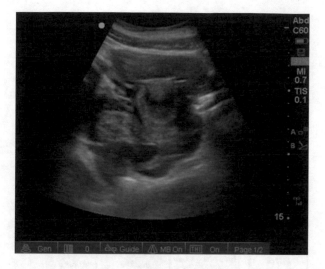

For hemodynamically unstable patients with suspected ruptured ectopic pregnancy, stabilization is the first priority. Volume resuscitation with isotonic intravenous fluids or blood products should be given as needed. Bedside ultrasonography of the pelvis along with a focused assessment with sonography for trauma (FAST) exam can aid in obtaining a diagnosis and expedite obstetric/gynecologic consultation [7]. The presumptive diagnosis of ruptured ectopic pregnancy can be made using the combination of a positive pregnancy test and evidence of free fluid in the abdomen with a bedside FAST exam or abdominal distention and peritonitis on exam (Fig. 1.1). Serum qualitative β-hCG levels may be easier to obtain and may return a faster result than a urine test or quantitative level. Unstable patients with ruptured ectopic pregnancies ultimately need surgery, and thus emergent obstetric/gynecologic consultation or transfer to a higher level of care center is necessary.

For hemodynamically stable patients, it is reasonable to obtain either a urine or blood qualitative β-hCG test before pursuing further work-up to confirm pregnancy. For the patient with a positive pregnancy test, transabdominal ultrasonography (TAUS) and transvaginal ultrasonography (TVUS) are the diagnostic modes of choice (see Fig. 1.2 for suggested algorithm). The authors begin with TAUS and, if indeterminate, proceed to TVUS. If bedside ultrasonography is available and the clinician is qualified, this will likely expedite the patient's disposition [8]. See Chap. 2 for a detailed discussion on the use of point-of-care ultrasound in the ED. If not, a radiology study can be performed. The initial goal is to determine whether or not an intrauterine pregnancy (IUP) is present. A yolk sac is the first definite sonographic sign of an IUP and can be visualized using TVUS beginning around the 5th week of pregnancy. If an IUP is confirmed, management is expectant. If no IUP is seen, further ultrasound characteristics can either raise or lower the suspicion for ectopic pregnancy. Ultrasound findings such as ectopic fetal pole or cardiac activity are diagnostic of an ectopic gestation, while other findings such as an adnexal mass or free pelvic fluid are concerning for an ectopic pregnancy

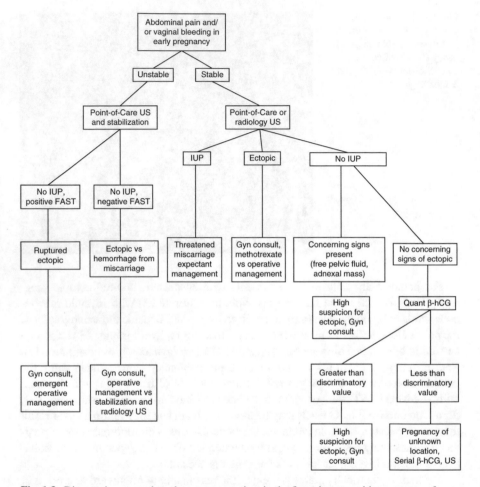

Fig. 1.2 Diagnostic approach to the pregnant patient in the first trimester with symptoms of abdominal pain and/or vaginal bleeding

(Fig. 1.3). One study reported a five times increased rate of ectopic pregnancy in patients with abnormal fluid in the cul-de-sac [9]. Abnormal free fluid has been described as any echogenic fluid or fluid that tracks more than one third up the posterior uterine wall [9] (Fig. 1.4).

A quantitative β-hCG level should also be obtained if an IUP is not visualized. There has been recent controversy in the literature regarding the "discriminatory zone," or the β-hCG level at which an IUP, if present, should be seen consistently by ultrasound. For TVUS, the discriminatory zone has traditionally been accepted as between 1000 and 2000 mIU/mL. If the β-hCG level is above this threshold and an IUP is not visualized, ectopic pregnancy should be strongly suspected. Multiple studies have sought to establish an exact β-hCG level at which there is higher clinical suspicion for ectopic pregnancy when TVUS is non-diagnostic. Some studies suggest that a β-hCG level lower than 1000–1500 mIU/mL increases suspicion,

Fig. 1.3 Transabdominal ultrasound showing a twin ectopic pregnancy in the right adnexa with surrounding free fluid

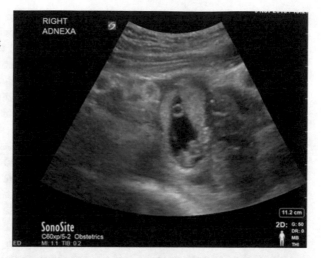

Fig. 1.4 Transvaginal ultrasound showing a left adnexal cyst and concomitant free fluid present in the posterior cul-de-sac

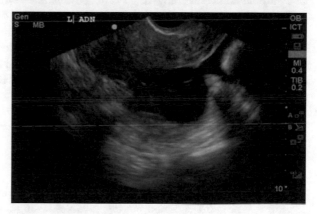

while other studies have failed to support a lower cutoff point [1, 3, 10]. Still other studies have shown that a normal pregnancy is possible well above the discriminatory zone, even if an IUP is not yet visualized on TVUS [11–13]. Therefore, caution should be used when interpreting a single β-hCG level. The authors recommend an ultrasound for all patients, regardless of β-hCG level [14]. There is no β-hCG level at which an ectopic pregnancy can be completely excluded. Serum quantitative β-hCG level is often not needed in the ED if the ultrasound shows an IUP.

For patients with no visualized IUP and ultrasound features either diagnostic or highly concerning for ectopic, the authors recommend obtaining a serum quantitative β-hCG level, as well as a complete blood count (CBC) and type and screen. Obstetric/gynecologic consultation is needed for aide in disposition, as hemodynamically stable patients with ectopic pregnancy may be candidates for methotrexate therapy instead of the historically standard laparoscopy and salpingectomy. The traditional operative approach has largely been replaced by the use of methotrexate in this patient population, based on several studies confirming the efficacy and safety of this modality [7, 15]. Several different methotrexate treatment protocols are available, with the single-dose protocol currently being most popular. The dose is 1 mg/kg or 50 mg/m² intramuscular (IM) [16]. For patients who are discharged after receiving methotrexate, they should be instructed to return on days 4 and 7 after administration for repeat β-hCG levels. It must be emphasized that patients are still at risk for rupture during treatment with methotrexate. In addition, all patients with an ectopic pregnancy who are Rh negative should be treated with rhesus immune globulin (RhIG), regardless of whether or not their initial presentation included vaginal bleeding [7].

After their initial ED workup, many patients will have a diagnosis of pregnancy of unknown location (PUL) based on a non-diagnostic ultrasound without signs concerning for ectopic. In hemodynamically stable patients with PUL, it is appropriate to repeat β-hCG measurement and consider repeat TVUS in 48 hours instead of initiating medical or surgical intervention for possible ectopic pregnancy. A rise of the β-hCG level greater than 50% is reassuring of a normal pregnancy, but is not diagnostic of an IUP [4, 7]. A slight rise, decrease, or stagnation of the β-hCG level is abnormal and concerning, as 71% of these women will eventually be diagnosed with ectopic pregnancy [6]. A significant drop in the β-hCG level is suggestive of miscarriage. Patients need to understand the importance of close follow-up and should return to the ED for repeat testing if their obstetrician cannot see them. More recent literature suggests that if the follow-up visit is non-diagnostic, a third visit on day 4 or day 7 following the initial visit for serial β-hCG testing can further minimize the risk of missing an ectopic pregnancy [17].

Heterotopic Pregnancies

Heterotopic pregnancy refers to simultaneous pregnancies in at least two different locations. The most common pairing involves a single IUP and an ectopic pregnancy, most commonly in a fallopian tube. Heterotopic pregnancies pose significant challenges to practitioners due to their rarity and difficulty in diagnosis; they also carry significant morbidity to patients. The incidence of heterotopic pregnancies has been previously reported to be approximately 1 in 30,000 pregnancies [18]. However, recently the incidence has been reported to be much greater, as high as 1 in 4,000–8,000 in the general population [19]. In individuals using assisted reproductive technologies (ART), the incidence is reported to be 1 in 100 pregnancies, making it a not uncommon clinical scenario [20]. Risk factors for heterotopic pregnancies include ART, prior ectopic pregnancy, prior tubal surgery or other tubal pathology, and history of pelvic inflammatory disease. Specifically, patients undergoing hormonal treatment for pregnancy, in vitro fertilization, intrauterine insemination, and those with tubal disease appear to be at the highest risk [21]. In a case series of 13 heterotopic pregnancies, six resulted from ovulation induction, six resulted from in vitro fertilization, and one occurred spontaneously [22].

Patients with heterotopic pregnancies can present similarly to those with threatened miscarriages and ectopic pregnancies. Symptoms include abdominal pain, vaginal bleeding, enlarged uterus, peritoneal irritation, and shock. However, the diagnosis is frequently missed. In a review of seven heterotopic pregnancies described in emergency medicine literature, none were diagnosed correctly upon the initial ED visit [23]. In patients with heterotopic pregnancies, the symptoms of the ectopic pregnancy can be mistakenly attributed to the intrauterine gestation once it is identified. To further complicate the diagnosis, the patient may have no symptoms, as approximately 50% of patients are asymptomatic [24].

Making the diagnosis of heterotopic pregnancy begins with obtaining a pregnancy test and a TVUS. Serum β-hCG levels are difficult to interpret in heterotopic pregnancies as the IUP can cause an appropriate rise in hormone levels. Often the diagnosis hinges on the clinician identifying possible heterotopic pregnancy risk factors. In a patient with risk factors for heterotopic pregnancy, especially the use of ART, close attention must be paid to the entire pelvis on ultrasound, even if an IUP is seen. Ultrasound findings that should prompt concern include free fluid, adnexal masses, ovarian cysts, hydrosalpinx, or significant pain with the examination (Fig. 1.5). Large free fluid in the pelvis should raise suspicion for a pathologic process. In patients undergoing ovulation stimulation, it can be difficult to distinguish between ascites from ovarian hyperstimulation syndrome and hemoperitoneum. Interpreting adnexal structures is also often difficult. Corpus luteum cysts can present with similar symptoms as ectopic pregnancy. Non-intrauterine cystic structures surrounded by echogenic rings have been shown to carry a high likelihood of pathology [25]. Somers et al. describe a case of heterotopic pregnancy in a woman without risk factors initially diagnosed as having an intrauterine pregnancy and ruptured corpus luteum cyst as the cause of her pain, who became unstable and was subsequently diagnosed with a ruptured ectopic pregnancy during emergency surgery. This case serves to illustrate challenge in diagnosis and the importance of remembering heterotopic pregnancy in the differential diagnosis [26].

Making an early diagnosis of heterotopic pregnancy has been shown to improve the chance of successfully carrying the intrauterine pregnancy to term. In a case series of 132 heterotopic pregnancies, 122 were diagnosed by ultrasound. Ultrasound findings in these patients included pelvic fluid (75%), hydrosalpinx (39%), uterine fluid (38%), and ovarian hyperstimulation syndrome (2.5%) [24]. In these patients,

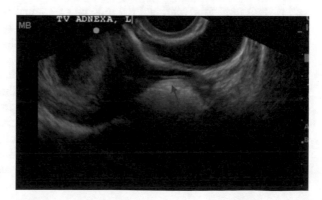

Fig. 1.5 Transvaginal ultrasound showing both an intrauterine pregnancy and hydrosalpinx, concerning for heterotopic

90 delivered live infants and 32 women suffered miscarriages (spontaneously, post-operatively, and late). Of the ten women with heterotopic pregnancies who were not diagnosed via ultrasound but rather later during surgery, only three women delivered live infants [24].

The management of heterotopic pregnancies includes aggressive resuscitation of clinically unstable patients and early obstetric consultation to discuss medical versus surgical management depending on the clinical scenario. If the patient is unstable and shows sign of shock, exploratory laparotomy or laparoscopy is indicated [22]. In stable patients, multiple treatment options exist including sonographic-guided aspiration and in situ injection of methotrexate, potassium chloride, or hyperosmolar glucose [27, 28].

First Trimester Miscarriages

Vaginal bleeding in pregnancy can complicate up to 20% of pregnancies and is a common complaint seen in the ED [29]. Spontaneous miscarriage (abortion) is defined as pregnancy loss before 20 weeks gestation and remains the most common complication of early pregnancy. Rates of subsequent fetal loss after a documented live IUP in the setting of a threatened miscarriage vary from 2.3% to as high as 14.3% [30].

Fetal abnormalities represent the largest cause of spontaneous miscarriage [31]. Many studies reflect that most miscarriages are due to fetal chromosomal abnormalities, but they can also result from placental abnormalities and maternal disease [32]. Other risk factors for miscarriage include previous miscarriages, advanced maternal age, and cigarette smoking. Maternal age has been reported to be a leading risk factor for spontaneous abortion. Studies have shown that increasing maternal age directly correlates with increasing rates of miscarriage, ranging from 9% at age 20 to 80% at age 45 [33]. The risk of miscarriage also increases significantly with the number of prior consecutive miscarriages.

Patients undergoing a spontaneous miscarriage may present with abdominal pain, vaginal bleeding, or they may be asymptomatic. The description of the pain varies from mild to severe, and the amount of vaginal bleeding may vary from a small amount of spotting to frank hemorrhage. Vaginal bleeding is common in the first trimester, and the amount of bleeding does not predict whether or not a miscarriage will ultimately occur.

Diagnosing a first trimester miscarriage involves performing a pelvic exam, laboratory studies, and imaging. During the pelvic exam, the clinician should seek to determine the size of the uterus and quantity of the vaginal bleeding and to assess for cervical dilatation. In a singleton pregnancy, the uterus should be contained in the pelvis during the first trimester. At 12 weeks' gestation, the fundal height should reach the pubic symphysis. The amount of bleeding should be ascertained and the patient resuscitated as needed. The cervical os should also be assessed either by direct visualization using a speculum or via digital examination during bimanual exam. Once a pelvic exam is performed and the patient is determined to be stable, an ultrasound should be performed.

Ultrasound is the most important step in diagnosing a first trimester miscarriage. Multiple studies exist which demonstrate the capability of emergency physicians to perform bedside ultrasounds in the evaluation of first trimester pregnancy [34–37]. The examination may begin as a transabdominal ultrasound and progress to a transvaginal ultrasound as needed. After an IUP has been confirmed, the most important factor to identify is the presence or absence of fetal cardiac activity. Cardiac activity can usually be visualized between 5.5 and 6 weeks' gestation. If fetal cardiac activity is not seen, then correlation between dating using crown rump length should be made to determine whether cardiac activity is expected. If no cardiac activity is seen, discussion with obstetrics is warranted, so arrangements may be made for further care. The presence of subchorionic hematomas has been shown to increase the chance of subsequent miscarriage, with rates ranging from 8.9 to 17.6%, with the greatest risk in women with large hematomas [38]. Other findings which have been associated with subsequent pregnancy loss include abnormally shaped yolk sacs and slow fetal heart rates.

In any pregnant patient with vaginal bleeding, the clinician must determine the patient's Rh status. Women who are Rh negative should be given RhIG. In the first trimester, one 50 mcg intramuscular dose is sufficient prophylaxis to prevent Rh alloimmunization, but there is no harm in giving the 300 mcg dose which is more readily available. While a serum β-hCG quantitative test is most useful in the ED when evaluating a PUL and less useful when a patient has an IUP, obtaining a quantitative β-hCG level may help facilitate outpatient care as obstetricians frequently trend β-hCG levels over time following a miscarriage. A CBC should be ordered to evaluate for significant anemia resulting from the bleeding. Most women with a first trimester pregnancy should also have a urinalysis performed as urinary tract infections have been shown to increase pregnancy complications including risk for miscarriage [39].

Once the appropriate physical exam, ultrasound, and lab findings are combined, the patient can then be placed into one of the differing categories of possible miscarriages (Table 1.1). A threatened miscarriage is defined as vaginal bleeding in pregnancy less than 20 weeks gestation with a closed cervical os. Many clinicians also include patients experiencing abdominal pain in early pregnancy with a closed cervical os and currently viable pregnancy in this definition. An inevitable miscarriage

Table 1.1 Definitions of types of miscarriages

Terminology	Definition
Threatened miscarriage	Vaginal bleeding (abdominal pain) with live IUP and closed cervical os
Inevitable miscarriage	Vaginal bleeding (abdominal pain) with live IUP and open cervical os
Incomplete miscarriage	Incomplete passage of products of conception
Complete miscarriage	Passage of all products of conception
Missed miscarriage	Fetal demise and no passage of products of conception
Septic miscarriage	Signs of both miscarriage and infection

is defined as vaginal bleeding in pregnancy less than 20 weeks gestation with a dilated cervical os. An incomplete miscarriage refers to the partial passage of products of conception, with remaining products present in the uterus. In a complete miscarriage, all of the products of conception have been passed. A pregnancy with fetal loss but no passage of tissue for 4 weeks is referred to as a missed miscarriage. Finally, a septic miscarriage refers to any miscarriage with signs of infection.

Hemodynamically stable patients diagnosed with a threatened miscarriage may be safely discharged home once close follow-up is established. Management for these patients is expectant. A complete miscarriage can be diagnosed in a patient with a previously documented live intrauterine pregnancy that now presents with vaginal bleeding and no remaining products of conception visualized in the uterus on ultrasound (empty uterus). If bleeding is controlled, patients with complete miscarriage may be discharged with close obstetric follow-up. In patients with heavy vaginal bleeding and septic miscarriage or if the diagnosis of complete versus incomplete miscarriage is unclear, obstetric consultation is indicated. For stable patients with incomplete or missed miscarriages, discussion with an obstetrician to arrange timely follow-up is appropriate. Patients with a missed miscarriage may be managed surgically with dilation and curettage or medically with misoprostol. If stable, they may be discharged to follow-up with obstetrics. Patients who are unstable, have significant bleeding, or who show signs of infection will require inpatient care on an obstetric service.

Complications of Assisted Reproductive Technologies (ART)

The use of assisted reproductive technologies (ART) to achieve pregnancy is becoming increasingly popular. It is estimated that 1% of pregnancies in the United States and 1–3% of pregnancies in the United Kingdom are the result of a procedure that falls under the umbrella of ART [40, 41]. ART have been associated with higher risks to the fetus even in singleton pregnancies when compared to non-ART pregnancies [42]. In vitro fertilization and intracytoplasmic sperm injection are the procedures most commonly associated with increased risks. Declining fertility both with and without ART is also associated with adverse perinatal outcomes such as low birth weight, preterm birth, and placental complications [43].

In addition to the risks associated with multiple gestational pregnancies as a result of multiple embryo transfers, patients who undergo ART are at increased risk of having an ectopic or heterotopic pregnancy [41]. The reported rates of ectopic pregnancy within the ART population vary widely, with rates as high as 8.6% [44]. As awareness increased about the risks of multiple gestations, doctors began to limit multiple embryo transfer, and thus the ectopic pregnancy incidence rate decreased in the 2000s [44]. Recent studies have also shown that ART without ovarian hyperstimulation decreases the ectopic risk [45, 46]. When an ectopic pregnancy does occur, the ectopic can be treated similarly to non-ART-associated ectopic pregnancies. If the

Fig. 1.6 Transabdominal ultrasound showing the presence of a hyperstimulated ovary showing multiple enlarged follicles

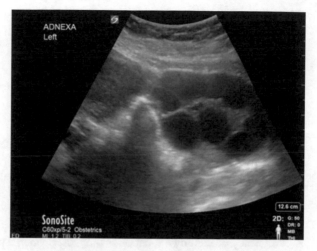

patient is appropriate for methotrexate therapy, it is equally effective, but there is a higher chance of needing two treatments to achieve successful resolution [47].

One additional complication of ART that can occur with or without a pregnancy is ovarian hyperstimulation syndrome (OHSS). OHSS occurs in 1% of women who receive exogenous gonadotropins as part of ART and should be considered in any patient undergoing ART who may or may not be pregnant as a result of their most recent cycle. OHSS occurs when there is a heightened response to increased gonadotropins, but the exact pathophysiology is not fully understood. The current understanding is that resultant increase in vascular permeability leads to third spacing of fluid, which can result in symptoms that range from mild (ovarian enlargement, abdominal pain, and bloating) to moderate (edema, ascites) to life threatening (severe end organ damage, profound hypotension, acute respiratory distress syndrome). In addition, enlarged ovaries in any stage of OHSS can put patients at increased risk for ovarian torsion or cyst rupture and hemorrhage [48]. Patients who have OHSS and are concurrently pregnant have a higher chance of pregnancy loss that is proportional to their degree of symptoms [49]. A diagnosis of OHSS can be made based on pelvic ultrasonography (Fig. 1.6). Treatment and disposition of these patients should be made in consultation with the reproductive endocrinologist who is overseeing their ART treatments and care.

Summary

Women commonly present to the ED with abdominal pain and vaginal bleeding in early pregnancy. First trimester complications include ectopic pregnancy, heterotopic pregnancy, and miscarriage. At a minimum, these complications are emotionally distressing to patients and may impact future fertility. Some complications such as ectopic and heterotopic pregnancy can be life threatening and are often missed on initial ED presentation. ART is becoming increasingly popular to achieve pregnancy, and emergency clinicians must be familiar with complications commonly associated with these treatments.

Key Points

- All women of childbearing age presenting to the ED with vaginal bleeding or abdominal pain should have a pregnancy test.
- Ruptured ectopic pregnancy is an obstetric emergency and should be considered in any female patient of reproductive age with unstable vital signs.
- There is no quantitative β-hCG level that can exclude ectopic pregnancy on the first visit.
- Pregnancy of unknown location is diagnosed when a patient has a positive pregnancy test, and no IUP or signs of ectopic pregnancy are visualized on ultrasound.
- Heterotopic pregnancy should be considered in any patient with an IUP and other concerning ultrasound findings such as free fluid or an adnexal mass.
- Miscarriages can often be managed expectantly as an outpatient.
- The use of assisted reproductive technologies dramatically increases a patient's risk of ectopic or heterotopic pregnancy.

References

1. Deutchman M, Tubay AT, Turok D. First trimester bleeding. Am Fam Physician. 2009;79:985–94.
2. Crochet JR, Bastian LA, Chireau MV. Does this woman have an ectopic pregnancy? The rational clinical examination systematic review. JAMA. 2013;309:1722–9.
3. Kohn MA, Kerr K, Malkevich D, et al. Beta-human chorionic gonadotropin levels and the likelihood of ectopic pregnancy in emergency department patients with abdominal pain or vaginal bleeding. Acad Emerg Med. 2003;10:119–26.
4. Marion LL, Meeks GR. Ectopic pregnancy: history, incidence, epidemiology, and risk factors. Clin Obstet Gynecol. 2012;55:376–86.
5. Bouyer J, Coste J, Shojael T, et al. Risk factors for ectopic pregnancy: a comprehensive analysis based on a large case-control, population-based study in France. Am J Epidemiol. 2003;157:185–94.
6. Barhart KT. Ectopic pregnancy. N Engl J Med. 2009;361:379–87.
7. Houry D, Keadey M. Complications in pregnancy part I: early pregnancy. Emerg Med Pract. 2007;9(6):1–28.
8. Mateer JR, Valley VT, Aiman EJ, et al. Outcome analysis of a protocol including bedside endovaginal sonography in patients at risk for ectopic pregnancy. Ann Emerg Med. 1996;27:283–9.
9. Dart R, McLean S, Dart L. Isolated fluid in the cul-de-sac: how well does it predict ectopic pregnancy? Am J Obstet Gynecol. 2000;185:522.

10. Kaplan BC, Dart RG, Moskos M, et al. Ectopic pregnancy: prospective study with improved diagnostic accuracy. Ann Emerg Med. 1996;28:10–7.
11. Wang R, Reynolds TA, West HH, et al. Use of a β-hCG discriminatory zone with bedside pelvic ultrasonography. Ann Emerg Med. 2011;58:12–20.
12. Doubilet PM, Benson CB, Bourne T, et al. Diagnostic criteria for nonviable pregnancy early in the first trimester. N Engl J Med. 2013;369:1443–51.
13. Ko JK, Cheung VY. Time to revisit the human chorionic gonadotropin discriminatory level in the management of pregnancy of unknown location. J Ultrasound Med. 2014;33:465–71.
14. Hahn SA, Lavonas EJ, Mace SE, et al. Clinical policy: critical issues in the initial evaluation and management of patients presenting to the emergency department in early pregnancy. Ann Emerg Med. 2012;60:381–90.
15. Varma R, Gupta J. Tubal ectopic pregnancy. BMJ Clin Evid. 2012;02:1406.
16. Celik H, Tosun M, Isik Y, et al. The role of early determination of beta-human chorionic gonadotropin levels in predicting the success of single-dose methotrexate treatment in ectopic pregnancy. Ginekol Pol. 2016;87:484–7.
17. Zee J, Sammel MD, Chung K, et al. Ectopic pregnancy prediction in women with a pregnancy of unknown location: data beyond 48 h are necessary. Hum Reprod. 2014;29:441–7.
18. Devoe R, Pratt J. Simultaneous intrauterine and extrauterine pregnancy. Am J Obstet Gynecol. 1948;56:1119–26.
19. Reece E, Petrie R, Sirmans M, Finster M, Todd W. Combined intrauterine and extrauterine gestations: a review. Am J Obstet Gynecol. 1983;146:323–30.
20. Goldman GA, Fisch B, Ovadia J, Tadir Y. Heterotopic pregnancy after assisted reproductive technologies. Obstet Gynecol Surv. 1992;47:217–21.
21. Tal J, Haddad S, Gordon N, Timor-Tritsch I. Heterotopic pregnancy after ovulation induction and assisted reproductive technologies: a literature review from 1971 to 1993. Fertil Steril. 1996;66:1.
22. Louis-Sylvestre C, Morice P, Chapron C, Dubuisson JB. Case report: the role of laparoscopy in the diagnosis and management of heterotopic pregnancies. Hum Reprod. 1997;12(5):1100–2.
23. Press GM, Martinez A. Heterotopic pregnancy diagnosed by emergency ultrasound. J Emerg Med. 2007;33(1):25–7.
24. Li XH, Ouyang Y, Lu GX. Value of transvaginal sonography in diagnosing heterotopic pregnancy after in-vitro fertilization with embryo transfer. Ultrasound Obstet Gynecol. 2013;41:563–9.
25. Dart RG. Role of pelvic ultrasonography in evaluation of symptomatic first-trimester pregnancy. Ann Emerg Med. 1999;33:310–20.
26. Somers M, Spears M, Maynard A, Syverud S. Ruptured heterotopic pregnancy presenting with relative bradycardia in a woman not receiving reproductive assistance. Ann Emerg Med. 2004;43:382–5.
27. Divry V, et al. Case of progressive intrauterine twin pregnancy after surgical treatment of cornual pregnancy. Fertil Steril. 2007;87(1):190.e1–3.
28. Wang Y, et al. Efficacy of local aspiration in the conservative treatment of live interstitial pregnancy coexisting with live intrauterine pregnancy after in vitro fertilization and embryo transfer. Chin Med J (Engl). 2012;25:1345–8.
29. Everett C. Incidence and outcome of bleeding before the 20th week of pregnancy: prospective study from general practice. BMJ. 1997;315:32–4.
30. Mohammed F. The outcome of pregnancies in 182 with threatened miscarriage. Arch Gynecol Obstet. 2004;270:86–90.
31. Hsu LYF. Prenatal diagnosis of chromosomal abnormalities through amniocentesis. In: Milunsky A, editor. Genetic disorders and the fetus. 4th ed. Baltimore: The Johns Hopkins University Press; 1998. p. 179.
32. Menasha J. Incidence and spectrum of chromosome abnormalities in spontaneous abortions: new insights from a 12-year study. Genet Med. 2005;7:251–63.
33. Nybo Andersen AM, Wohlfahrt J, Christes P, et al. Maternal age and fetal loss: population based register linkage study. BMJ. 2000;320–1708.

34. Blavias M, Sierzenski P, Plecque D, et al. Do emergency physicians save time when locating a live intrauterine pregnancy with bedside ultrasonography? Acad Emerg Med. 2000;9:988.
35. Adhikari S, Blavias M, Lyon M. Diagnosis and management of ectopic pregnancy using bedside transvaginal ultrasonography in the ED: a 2-year experience. Am J Emerg Med. 2007;6:591–6.
36. Varner C, Balaban D, McLeod S, et al. Fetal outcomes following emergency department point-of-care ultrasound for vaginal bleeding in early pregnancy. Can Fam Physician. 2016;7:572–8.
37. Chiem AT, Chan CH, Ibrahim DY, et al. Pelvic ultrasonography and length of stay in the ED: an observational study. Am J Emerg Med. 2014;12:1464–9.
38. Tuuli MG. Perinatal outcomes in women with subchorionic hematoma: a systematic review and meta-analysis. Obstet Gynecol. 2001;117:1205–12.
39. Glaser AP, Schaeffer AJ. Urinary tract infection and bacteriuria in pregnancy. Urol Clin North Am. 2015;4:547–60.
40. Society for Assisted Reproductive Technology, American Society for Reproductive Medicine. Assisted reproductive technology in the United States: 2001 results generated from the American Society for Reproductive Medicine/Society for Assisted Reproductive Technology registry. Fertil Steril. 2007;87:1253–66.
41. Land JA, Evers JL. Risks and complications in assisted reproductive techniques: report of an ESHRE consensus meeting. Hum Reprod. 2003;18:455–7.
42. Qin J, Liu X, Sheng X, et al. Assisted reproductive technology and the risk of pregnancy-related complications and adverse pregnancy outcomes in singleton pregnancies: a meta-analysis of cohort studies. Fertil Steril. 2016;105:73–85.
43. Luke B, Gopal D, Cabral H, et al. Perinatal outcomes of singleton siblings: the effects of changing maternal fertility status. J Assis Reprod Genet. 2016. [Epub ahead of print]
44. Perkins KM, Boulet SL, Kissin DM, et al. Risk of ectopic pregnancy associated with assisted reproductive technology in the United States, 2001-2011. Obstet Gynecol. 2015;125:70–8.
45. Bu Z, Xiong Y, Wang K, et al. Risk factors for ectopic pregnancy in assisted reproductive technology: a 6-year, single-center study. Fertil Steril. 2016. [Epub ahead of print]
46. Londra L, Moreau C, Strobino D, et al. Ectopic pregnancy after in vitro fertilization: differences between fresh and frozen-thawed cycles. Fertil Steril. 2015;104:110–8.
47. Ohannessian A, Crochet P, Courbiere B, et al. Methotrexate treatment for ectopic pregnancy after assisted reproductive technology: a case-control study. Gynecol Obstet Fertil. 2016;44:341–4.
48. Kwik M, Maxwell E. Pathophysiology, treatment and prevention of ovarian hyperstimulation syndrome. Curr Opin Obstet Gynecol. 2016;28:236–41.
49. Raziel A, Friedler S, Schachter M, et al. Increased early pregnancy loss in IVF patients with severe ovarian hyperstimulation syndrome. Hum Reprod. 2002;17:107–11.

Chapter 2
Emergency Department Ultrasound in Pregnancy

Cory Wittrock and Erica Peethumnongsin

Introduction

Pregnant patients often present to the emergency department (ED) with complaints of abdominal pain and vaginal bleeding, particularly in the first trimester. Point-of-care ultrasound is a useful tool for rapid assessment of the pregnant ED patient, allowing emergency physicians to quickly diagnose unstable conditions like ectopic pregnancy (pregnancy outside of the uterus) at the bedside. While obstetricians employ comprehensive ultrasound imaging for a variety of purposes, such as dating or detection of fetal anomalies, the goals of point-of-care ultrasound are limited by design. These studies seek to quickly, but accurately, answer very focused questions and, by necessity, must be narrow in scope. Point-of-care ultrasound can be used for identifying early pregnancy location (intrauterine vs. ectopic vs. indeterminate), gestational dating, and limited fetal biometry.

Image Acquisition

Ultrasound images in early pregnancy can be acquired in two ways, transabdominally and transvaginally. Transvaginal ultrasound (TVUS) is more sensitive due to the probe's proximity to the uterus, but it requires placement of a sterile probe cover, emptying of the bladder, and appropriate positioning of the patient. Transabdominal

C. Wittrock, M.D. (✉)
Department of Emergency Medicine, MedStar Georgetown University Hospital,
3800 Reservoir Road NW, Washington, DC 20007, USA
e-mail: corywittrock@gmail.com

E. Peethumnongsin, M.D.
Division of Emergency Medicine, Department of Surgery, Duke University Hospital,
2301 Erwin Road, Durham, NC 27710, USA

© Springer International Publishing AG 2017
J. Borhart (ed.), *Emergency Department Management of Obstetric Complications*,
DOI 10.1007/978-3-319-54410-6_2

ultrasound (TAUS), by comparison, is faster and easier but provides lower-resolution images, so very early intrauterine gestations may not be detectable by this method. The authors recommend using TAUS as the initial imaging modality in all pregnant patients because it is less invasive, but inconclusive TAUS should be followed by TVUS.

Transabdominal Technique

TAUS is best performed with a low-frequency (2–5 MHz) curvilinear probe because of the wide footprint and deep tissue penetration. Because the probe is distant from the tissues of interest, imaging improves with a full bladder because this fluid provides a good acoustic medium for ultrasound wave propagation. With any point-of-care ultrasound, the authors adhere to the convention of orienting the probe with the indicator either toward the patient's right side or toward the patient's head. For transverse (axial/coronal) TAUS views, the probe should be oriented to the patient's right and placed in the suprapubic region of the abdomen at midline as shown in Fig. 2.1. The probe should then fan superiorly and inferiorly to obtain a complete view of the uterus (Fig. 2.2).

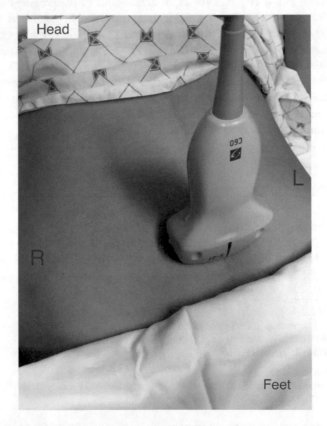

Fig. 2.1 Transabdominal ultrasound, transverse view. Note probe orientation with dot indicator (*) to patient's right side

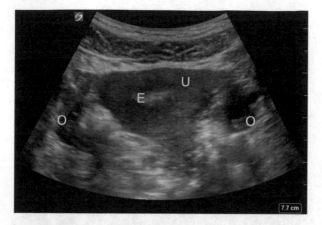

Fig. 2.2 TAUS transverse view. The uterus (U) is seen in the center of the image with its hyper-echoic endometrial stripe (E). The ovaries (O) are seen laterally

Incomplete imaging of the uterus may miss important findings, such as twin gestations or free fluid. A longitudinal (sagittal) view of the uterus should also be obtained by orienting the probe vertically and fanning side to side (Fig. 2.3). This view is best for evaluating the cervix and endometrial stripe and may allow easier detection of free fluid in the cul-de-sac (Fig. 2.4).

Bilateral adnexal imaging in the transverse plane is also critical in early pregnancy, because the vast majority of ectopic pregnancies are located in the adnexa [1]. An adequate adnexal view should contain the uterus medially and the pelvic brim laterally, with the iliac vessels visualized between these structures (Fig. 2.5). The ovary and, if fluid filled, the fallopian tube may be seen in this area but are not always visible with TAUS due to the lower overall image resolution. If an intrauterine pregnancy (IUP) is detected, calculations of gestational age and fetal heart rate should also be performed. These techniques will be discussed later in more detail in the sections on dating and fetal biometry.

Transvaginal Technique

TVUS imaging provides greater detail than TAUS because the endocavitary probe has a higher frequency (5–8 MHz), allowing better imaging of more superficial structures, and is placed directly against the cervix by insertion into the vaginal canal. As mentioned earlier, TVUS requires the use of a sterile probe cover and sterile gel to protect the patient from contamination by the inserted probe. Because the probe lies against the cervix, a full bladder confers no benefit and can actually impair imaging by deflecting the uterus superiorly/posteriorly and away from the probe. For this reason, patients should empty their bladder immediately before TVUS. When inserting the probe, a common error is to advance too deeply and lodge the probe in the posterior fornix, preventing any view of a typical anteverted uterus. To avoid this, look to the screen immediately after probe insertion and

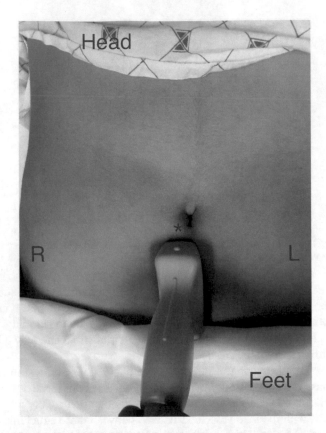

Fig. 2.3 Transabdominal ultrasound, longitudinal view. Note probe orientation with dot indicator (*) to patient's head

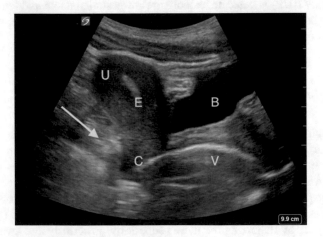

Fig. 2.4 TAUS longitudinal view. The uterus (U) is seen in the center of view with the hyperechoic endometrial stripe (E) and cervix (C) deep to the fundus. The anechoic bladder (B) is seen anteriorly to the vaginal vault (V). Note the potential space of the cul-de-sac (*arrow*), which can be replaced with free fluid

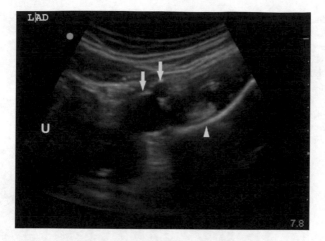

Fig. 2.5 TAUS adnexal view in the transverse plane. The region of interest is bordered by the uterus (U) medially and the pelvic brim (*arrowhead*) laterally, with the iliac vessels (*arrows*) located in between

Fig. 2.6 Endocavitary probe orientation, sagittal view. Note the probe dot indicator (*) is pointed superiorly to acquire sagittal views of the pelvis. The probe is swept horizontally left and right to image the pelvic organs

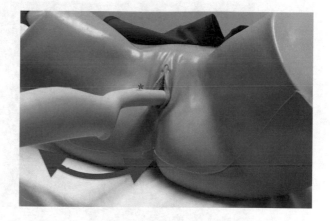

continue to watch the screen as you advance the probe. If there is difficulty locating the uterus after insertion, slowly pull back and/or adjust the angle of the probe. Positioning of the endocavitary probe is similar to the mechanics of a speculum exam and should be adjusted the same way. When in position, the probe indicator should be pointed either toward the ceiling (Fig. 2.6) or the patient's right by turning the probe in a counterclockwise direction (Fig. 2.7). For longitudinal, or sagittal, views, the indicator will be toward the ceiling and the probe will fan from side to side to visualize the entire uterus (Fig. 2.8). For transverse, or coronal, views, the probe indicator will be oriented to the patient's right and should fan anteriorly and posteriorly through the uterus (Fig. 2.9). Adnexal views are best obtained in the transverse orientation and are analogous to the TAUS adnexal views with the uterus located medially, the pelvic brim laterally, and the ovary and iliac vessels in between (Fig. 2.10).

Fig. 2.7 Endocavitary probe orientation, coronal view. Note the probe dot indicator (*) is pointed to the patient's right to acquire coronal views of the pelvis. The probe is swept superiorly and inferiorly to investigate the pelvic organs in the coronal view

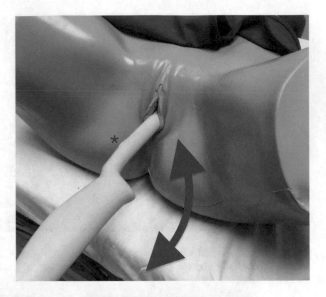

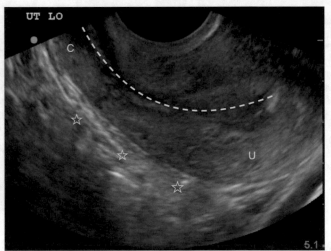

Fig. 2.8 TVUS longitudinal/sagittal view. The uterus (U) is seen closest to the endocavitary probe foot print. The cervix(C) is seen at the left of the image and the endometrial stripe (*dotted line*) traverses the uterus. Deep to the uterus is the cul-de-sac (*stars*), which should be investigated for anechoic free fluid

Fig. 2.9 TVUS transverse view. The right ovary (O) is visualized adjacent to the uterus (U). In this orientation, a limited view of the hyperechoic endometrial stripe (E) is also obtained

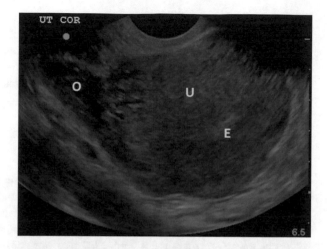

Fig. 2.10 TVUS adnexal view in the transverse plane. The left ovary (*star*) lies in its usual position lateral to the uterus (U) between the iliac vessels (*arrows*) and the pelvic brim (*arrowhead*)

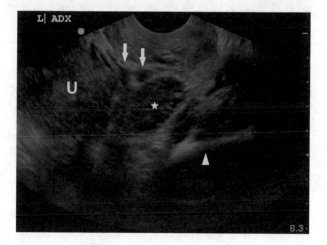

Application of Point-of-Care Ultrasound to the Pregnant Emergency Department Patient

Numerous studies have shown that with sufficient training, emergency physicians can use point-of-care ultrasound as a clinical tool for the rapid, bedside assessment of pregnant patients with the primary goal of determining pregnancy location— intrauterine, ectopic, or indeterminate (pregnancy of unknown location) [2–5].

Patients without demonstrated intrauterine gestations are at high risk for ectopic pregnancy, so early identification of these patients is crucial to providing timely, and sometimes lifesaving, care. On the other hand, detection of an intrauterine pregnancy can reassure, in the case of a stable patient, or direct efforts toward the diagnosis and management of a different condition in the unstable patient.

Intrauterine Pregnancy

The ultrasound finding easiest to interpret in early pregnancy is a normal intrauterine pregnancy (IUP). The authors define an IUP as a gestational sac containing, at a minimum, a yolk sac with or without the presence of an identifiable fetal pole. Historically, the presence of a double decidual sign (concentric hyperechoic and hypoechoic rings surrounding a fluid-filled sac) was considered the earliest sign of an IUP, but studies have shown this to be potentially deceptive, as this finding correlates poorly with actual presence of an IUP [6]. Therefore, the authors consider an empty sac within the uterus to be nondiagnostic, as discussed in more detail in the section on indeterminate location.

A yolk sac is the earliest sign of an IUP, detectable as early as the fifth week of gestation by TVUS, and appears as a circular structure within a fluid-filled sac, sometimes casually referred to as a "sac within a sac" or a "cheerio" due to its similarity to the breakfast cereal (Fig. 2.11) [7, 8]. Three to 4 days after the development of the yolk sac, a fetal pole can first be detected, with cardiac activity visible starting at 6 weeks [9]. At this early stage of pregnancy, a normal fetal pole will be immediately adjacent to the yolk sac, sometimes appearing contiguous with the sac's wall (Fig. 2.12). Of note, special consideration is necessary with patients using assisted reproductive technology because they are at much higher risk for heterotopic pregnancy (simultaneous IUP and ectopic pregnancy) than the general population (approximately 1 in 100 vs. 1 in 4000–30,000). These patients require comprehensive radiology imaging, even when an IUP is seen at the bedside [10–14].

Fig. 2.11 TVUS view with yolk sac (*arrow*)

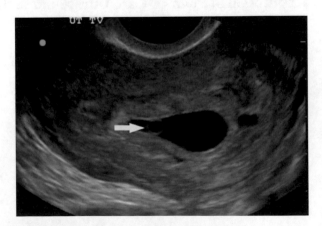

Fig. 2.12 TVUS view with yolk sac (*arrowhead*) and small adjacent fetal pole (*arrow*)

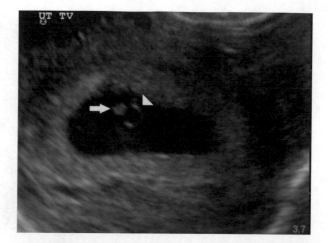

Fig. 2.13 TAUS view in the transverse plane with large ectopic pregnancy (*star*) visible in the left adnexa. A small pseudogestational sac (*arrow*) is seen within the uterus (U)

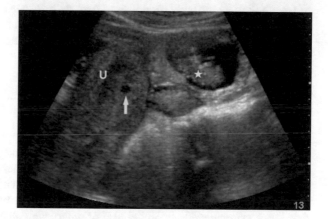

Ectopic Pregnancy

Although ectopic pregnancy should always be considered whenever an IUP is not detected, in some cases, the ectopic can be directly visualized using point-of-care ultrasound. For this reason, careful inspection of the adnexa is a vital component of any bedside exam. As discussed in the previous section, a fluid-filled sac within the uterus is not sufficient for diagnosis of an IUP because the hormonal changes that accompany pregnancy of any location may cause the development of intrauterine fluid collections, known as "pseudosacs," in up to 20% of ectopic pregnancies [15, 16]. Figure 2.13 shows an example of a large fetus in the left adnexa with a small pseudosac in the otherwise empty uterus that could have been mistaken for an IUP.

When an ectopic is detected (or suspected), additional focused assessment with sonography in trauma (FAST) views (right upper quadrant, left upper quadrant) of the abdomen should also be obtained to evaluate for free fluid (Fig. 2.14). Although a small amount of pelvic free fluid is common in normal pregnancies, the presence

Fig. 2.14 Right upper
quadrant FAST view from
a patient with a ruptured
ectopic demonstrating free
fluid (*star*) in Morison's
pouch between the liver
(L) and kidney (K)

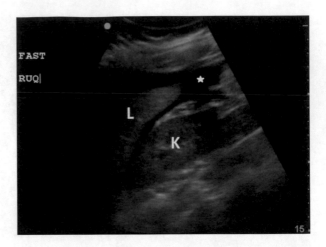

of free fluid in an unstable patient or patient with suspected ectopic should prompt
immediate OB/GYN consultation. The characteristics of the fluid are also important, as studies have shown that the presence of echogenic fluid is very sensitive for
the presence of hemoperitoneum [17, 18].

Pregnancy of Unknown Location

When no IUP is identified and a clear ectopic pregnancy is not detected, this is
defined as a pregnancy of unknown location (PUL). These patients may have normal pregnancies that have not yet developed to a stage that is visible by TVUS, may
be experiencing a spontaneous miscarriage, or they may have an ectopic pregnancy
that is not yet detectable by imaging. For emergency physicians, the greatest concern is an ectopic pregnancy; however, hasty designation of an abnormal pregnancy
without definitive proof may lead to the unnecessary disruption of an otherwise
viable pregnancy.

A great deal of study and debate has recently emerged surrounding the concept of
the discriminatory zone, and its utility has been called into question [19]. The discriminatory zone is the level of beta-hCG at which an IUP, if present, should be seen
consistently. For TVUS, the discriminatory zone is generally accepted as between
1000–2000 IU/mL. Previous practice was to use β-HCG levels to determine the utility of ultrasonography—i.e., levels below the discriminatory zone did not warrant
imaging because, presumably, no IUP was likely to be detected. Recent studies have
found fault with this practice. In one study, deferring imaging due to β-HCG levels
below the discriminatory threshold delayed diagnosis of ectopic pregnancy by more
than 5 days [20]. In another study, ectopic pregnancies were present in as many as
40% of patients with β-HCG levels below the discriminatory zone [21].

Using a discriminatory threshold to exclude a viable pregnancy is also problematic. Wang et al. [22] were unable to identify any β-HCG level above which 100% of IUPs could be visualized. Other studies have shown that normal intrauterine pregnancy is subsequently possible above the discriminatory zone, even if an IUP is not yet visualized on TVUS [23, 24]. Therefore, caution should be used when interpreting a single beta-hCG measurement. The current American College of Emergency Physicians (ACEP) clinical policy is to obtain or perform a pelvic ultrasound on all patients presenting in early pregnancy with abdominal pain or vaginal bleeding regardless of the β-HCG levels, which should not be used to defer imaging or rule out ectopic pregnancy [25]. There is no beta-hCG level in which an ectopic pregnancy can be completely ruled out. If the patient is hemodynamically stable, it is appropriate to repeat beta-hCG measurements and consider repeating TVUS in 48 hours instead of initiating treatment for possible ectopic pregnancy based on the discriminatory zone alone.

Secondary Applications of Point-of-Care Ultrasound in Early Pregnancy

Although the main objective of bedside ultrasonography in early pregnancy is the determination of pregnancy location, other useful information can be obtained with little additional effort. Comprehensive fetal assessment is beyond the scope of a point-of-care scan, but dating and measurement of cardiac activity are appropriate extensions of a limited bedside exam.

Fetal Gestational Dating

Because calculations of gestational age are more accurate early in pregnancy, these measurements are useful to patients and their obstetricians and should be obtained when possible. The crown-rump length (CRL) is the best method for dating within the first trimester and is accurate up to 14 weeks gestation [26–32]. As shown in Fig. 2.15, an appropriate CRL measurement is a straight line drawn from the crown of the head to the rump, taking care not to include limb buds or the yolk sac. For the most accurate measurement, adjust the probe to obtain a view of the fetus in its longest orientation.

When the patient has reached her second trimester, biparietal diameter (BPD) is the preferred dating measurement. This method is most accurate between 14 and 20 weeks gestation (±7 days within this window) but declines in accuracy as the pregnancy progresses beyond these dates [32–35]. An accurate BPD should be measured in the axial orientation in plane with the third ventricle and bilateral thalami by drawing a line from the innermost edge of the posterior calvarium to the outermost edge of the anterior calvarium (Fig. 2.16). This convention prevents exaggeration of

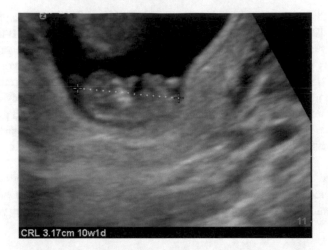

Fig. 2.15 Crown-rump length, TAUS image (zoomed in)

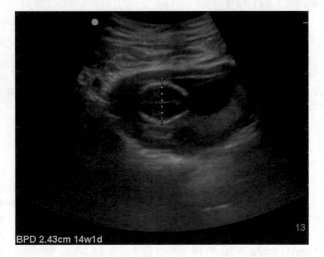

Fig. 2.16 Biparietal diameter, TAUS image

the measurement by acoustic enhancement of the posterior calvarium, an artifact that makes the calvarium's thickness appear greater and artificially increases the BPD.

Other methods can also be used for gestational dating in the second and third trimester, but are not as accurate as the BPD [36]. Examples include femur, tibia, or humerus length, in which the bone is captured in its longest orientation and the full length of the cortex is measured, or head or abdominal circumference, in which an appropriate axial view of the structure is outlined for calculation of the circumference.

On occasion, the BPD may be difficult to obtain due to fetal positioning, and femur length is an acceptable alternative, though this measurement may be off by as much as 1–3 weeks [29].

Fetal Biometry

In addition to dating, ultrasound is also useful for the detection and measurement of fetal cardiac activity. The first step is to look for the presence of cardiac movement, which may be detectable by TVUS as early as 6 weeks. Cardiac activity appears as a rhythmic flicker within the fetal pole in early gestations or varying degrees of cardiac anatomy in more advanced pregnancies. When this activity is detected, the next step is to measure the rate of activity, which can have prognostic value when abnormal. Normal fetal heart rates should be >100 beats per minute before 6.3 weeks or >120 bpm after 6.3 weeks; fetal bradycardia is associated with poor outcomes, including fetal loss [37]. Fetal tachycardia is typically defined as rates >160–180 bpm. The prognosis for fetal tachycardia is good, often resolving spontaneously without intervention [38].

To measure fetal heart rate, M-mode is used, which follows the changes in position of one portion of the image over time. The area of interest is first identified in the standard 2D B-mode. When M-mode is applied, a line appears on the screen and should be placed directly across the fetal heart. Activating M-mode measurement plots out the changes in position of the selected area over time, which looks like a series of horizontal lines and waves. Because the heart is moving, its position will change rhythmically and can be detected as a wavelike pattern. The rate can then be measured by placing the calipers at the same place on two consecutive waves, which represent cardiac cycles (Fig. 2.17). Due to concerns about the higher thermal energy used for spectral Doppler, the authors do not employ this method for measuring cardiac activity and recommend against its use [39, 40].

Summary

Point-of-care ultrasound is a useful tool for rapid assessment of the pregnant emergency department patient. Two methods can be used for image acquisition, transabdominal and transvaginal imaging, and must be employed whenever the location of the pregnancy is in doubt. The primary goal of bedside ultrasound in the pregnant patient is to identify an intrauterine pregnancy and an ectopic pregnancy or, when neither can be visualized, to designate a pregnancy of unknown location. In patients

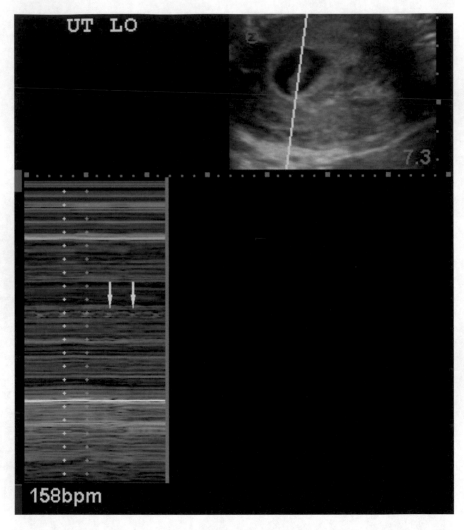

Fig. 2.17 Fetal heart rate measurement using M-mode. The 2D view is shown in the upper portion of the screen, while the M-mode output is below. The *dotted lines* are placed at two consecutive cycles (cycles emphasized by *arrows*) to calculate a rate of 158 bpm (*lower left*)

with hemodynamic compromise and in whom pretest probability for ectopic pregnancy is high, further evaluation for free fluid and prompt OB/GYN consultation should occur. There is no beta-hCG level at which an ectopic pregnancy can be completely ruled out, and ultrasound should be obtained in all patients presenting in early pregnancy with abdominal pain or vaginal bleeding. When possible, gestational dating and measurement of fetal heart rate should be performed to guide obstetric management.

Key Points

• Perform transabdominal imaging before proceeding to transvaginal imaging to prevent unnecessary TVUS.
• Intrauterine pregnancy is defined as a gestational sac containing, at a minimum, a yolk sac with or without the presence of an identifiable fetal pole. A gestational sac without a yolk sac and/or fetal pole may be a pseudosac and cannot exclude the presence of an ectopic pregnancy.
• Do not use β-HCG levels to rule in *or* rule out ectopic pregnancy—always get an ultrasound when pregnancy location is in doubt.
• Patients using assisted reproductive technology are at higher risk of heterotopic pregnancy and should undergo comprehensive radiology ultrasound if stable.
• Crown-rump length is measured for dating in the first trimester. Biparietal diameter is the preferred measurement in the second trimester and beyond.
• Measure fetal heart rate using M-mode—spectral Doppler confers a theoretical risk of thermal injury to the fetus.

References

1. Bouyer J, Coste J, Fernandez H, et al. Sites of ectopic pregnancy: a 10-year population-based study of 1800 cases. Hum Reprod. 2002;17(12):3224–30.
2. American College of Emergency Physicians. Policy statement: definition of clinical ultrasonography. Approved January 2014.
3. American Institute of Ultrasound in Medicine. AIUM officially recognizes ACEP emergency ultrasound guidelines. Sound Waves Newslett. Issue: November 17, 2011.
4. American College of Emergency Physicians. Policy statement: emergency ultrasound imaging criteria compendium. Ann Emerg Med. 2006;48:487–510.
5. Stein JC, Wang R, Adler N, et al. Emergency physician ultrasonography for evaluating patients at risk for ectopic pregnancy: a meta-analysis. Ann Emerg Med. 2010;56:674–83.
6. Doubilet PM, Benson CB. Double sac sign and intradecidual sign in early pregnancy: interobserver reliability and frequency of occurrence. J Ultrasound Med. 2013;32(7):1207–14.
7. Laing FC, Frates MC. Ultrasound evaluation during the first trimester of pregnancy. In: Callen PW, editor. Ultrasonography in obstetrics and gynecology. 4th ed. Philadelphia: WB Saunders Co; 2000.
8. Bree RL, Edwards M, Böhm-Vélez M, et al. Transvaginal sonography in the evaluation of normal early pregnancy: correlation with HCG level. Am J Roentgenol. 1989;153(1):75–9.
9. Noble VE, Nelson BP. First trimester ultrasound. In: Manual of emergency and critical care ultrasound. 2nd ed. Cambridge: Cambridge University Press; 2011.
10. Mukul LV, Teal SB. Current management of ectopic pregnancy. Obstet Gynecol Clin North Am. 2007;34:403–19.
11. Chin HY, Chen FP, Wang CJ, et al. Heterotopic pregnancy after in-vitro fertilization–embryo transfer. Int J Gynecol Obstet. 2004;86:411–6.
12. Reece EA, Petrie RH, Sirmans MF, et al. Combined intrauterine and extrauterine gestations: a review. Am J Obstet Gynecol. 1983;146:323–30.
13. Tal J, Haddad S, Gordon N, et al. Heterotopic pregnancy after ovulation induction and assisted reproductive technologies: a literature review from 1971 to 1993. Fertil Steril. 1996;66:1–12.

14. Inion I, Gerris J, Joostens M, et al. An unexpected triplet heterotopic pregnancy after replacement of two embryos. Hum Reprod. 1998;13:1999–2001.
15. Filly RA. Ectopic pregnancy: the role of sonography. Radiology. 1987;162:661.
16. Bhatt S, Ghazale H, Dogra VS. Sonographic evaluation of ectopic pregnancy. Radiol Clin North Am. 2007;45:549.
17. Nyberg DA, Hughes MP, Mack LA, et al. Extrauterine findings of ectopic pregnancy of transvaginal US: importance of echogenic fluid. Radiology. 1991;178(3):823–6.
18. Sickler GK, Chen PC, Dubinsky TJ, et al. Free echogenic pelvic fluid: correlation with hemoperitoneum. J Ultrasound Med. 1998;17(7):431–5.
19. Doubilet PM, Benson CB, Bourne T, et al. Diagnostic criteria for nonviable pregnancy early in the first trimester. N Engl J Med. 2013;369:1443–51.
20. Barnhart K, Mennuti MT, Benjamin I, et al. Prompt diagnosis of ectopic pregnancy in an emergency department setting. Obstet Gynecol. 1994;84(6):1010–5.
21. Kaplan BC, Dart RG, Moskos M, et al. Ectopic pregnancy: prospective study with improved diagnostic accuracy. Ann Emerg Med. 1996;28(1):10–7.
22. Wang R, Reynolds TA, West HH, et al. Use of a β-hCG discriminatory zone with bedside pelvic ultrasonography. Ann Emerg Med. 2011;58(1):12–20.
23. Ko JK, Cheung VY. Time to revisit the human chorionic gonadotropin discriminatory level in the management of pregnancy of unknown location. J Ultrasound Med. 2014;33:465–71.
24. Doubilet PM, Benson CB. Further evidence against the reliability of the human chorionic gonadotropin discriminatory level. J Ultrasound Med. 2011;30:1637–42.
25. Hahn SA, Lavonas EJ, Mace SE, et al. Clinical policy: Critical issues in the initial evaluation and management of patients presenting to the emergency department in early pregnancy. Ann Emerg Med. 2012;60(3):381–90.
26. Daya S. Accuracy of gestational age estimation by means of fetal crown-rump length measurement. Am J Obstet Gynecol. 1993;168(3):903–8.
27. Wisser J, Dirschedl P, Krone S. Estimation of gestational age by transvaginal sonographic measurement of greatest embryonic length in dated human embryos. Ultrasound Obstet Gynecol. 1994;4(6):457–62.
28. Robinson HP, Fleming JE. A critical evaluation of sonar "crown-rump length" measurements. Br J Obstet Gynaecol. 1975;82(9):702–10.
29. Butt K, Lim K. Society of Obstetricians and Gynaecologists of Canada. Determination of gestational age by ultrasound. J Obstet Gynaecol Can. 2014;36(2):171–83.
30. National Institute for Health and Clinical Excellence. Antenatal Care (CG62). Published March 2008, last updated March 2016. http://guidance.nice.org.uk/CG62.
31. Salomon LJ, Alfirevic Z, Bilardo CM, et al. ISUOG practice guidelines: performance of first-trimester fetal ultrasound scan. Ultrasound Obstet Gynecol. 2013;41(1):102–13.
32. American College of Obstetricians and Gynecologists. Committee opinion no 611: method for estimating due date. Obstet Gynecol. 2014;124(4):863–6.
33. Campbell S, Warsof SL, Little D, et al. Routine ultrasound screening for the prediction of gestational age. Obstet Gynecol. 1985;65(5):613–20.
34. Benson CB, Doubilet PM. Sonographic prediction of gestational age: accuracy of second- and third-trimester fetal measurements. Am J Roentgenol. 1991;157(6):1275–7.
35. Filly RA, Hadlock FP. Sonographic determination of menstrual age. In: Callen PW, editor. Ultrasonography in obstetrics and gynecology. 4th ed. Philadelphia: WB Saunders Co; 2000.
36. Hadlock FP. Sonographic estimation of fetal age and weight. Radiol Clin North Am. 1990;28(1):39–50.
37. Doubilet PM, Benson CB. Embryonic heart rate in the early first trimester: what rate is normal? J Ultrasound Med. 1995;14(6):431–4.
38. Lulić Jurjević R, Podnar T, Vesel S. Diagnosis, clinical features, management, and post-natal follow-up of fetal tachycardias. Cardiol Young. 2009;19(5):486–93.
39. American Institute of Ultrasound in Medicine. Official statement: statement on measurement of fetal heart rate. Approved November 5, 2011.
40. American Institute of Ultrasound in Medicine. Official statement: statement on the safe use of doppler ultrasound during 11–14 week scans (or earlier in pregnancy). Approved March 21, 2016.

Chapter 3
Approach to the Patient with Nausea and Vomiting in Pregnancy

Lindsey DeGeorge and Lauren Wiesner

Introduction

Nausea and vomiting is a common problem during pregnancy estimated to impact 70–80% of pregnancies [1]. The exact incidence is difficult to determine because many women do not seek medical attention. The primary treatment for these patients is supportive, and symptoms typically resolve by 14–16 weeks of pregnancy. Although nausea and vomiting contributes to maternal stress and decreased quality of life, it is generally not associated with adverse maternal or fetal outcomes. Nausea and vomiting of pregnancy does, however, represent a significant cost burden to the healthcare system, estimated to cost nearly 2 billion dollars in 2012 alone [2]. Rarely, nausea and vomiting is severe, resulting in weight loss, dehydration, and electrolyte disturbances. When this occurs, it is known as hyperemesis gravidarum (HG). Estimates regarding the prevalence of HG vary, but it is thought to affect between 0.5 and 2% of pregnancies, with some literature suggesting it occurs in up to 3% of pregnancies [3]. According to a recent Cochrane review, HG is the leading cause of hospital admissions in early pregnancy [4]. HG typically occurs between the 4th and 10th week of gestation but may occur at any point during pregnancy. The exact etiology of HG is unknown and is thought to be multifactorial. Factors thought to contribute to the pathogenesis of HG include gestational-induced hormonal changes, genetics, preexisting upper GI dysmotility, and *H. pylori* infection [5, 6]. HG is associated with higher risk of pregnancy complications and negative outcomes such as preterm birth, small-for-gestational-age infants, and low birth weight [6].

L. DeGeorge, M.D. • L. Wiesner, M.D. (✉)
Department of Emergency Medicine, MedStar Washington Hospital Center,
110 Irving St NW, Washington, DC 20010, USA
e-mail: degeorge.lindsey@gmail.com; lauren.m.wiesner@medstar.net

© Springer International Publishing AG 2017
J. Borhart (ed.), *Emergency Department Management of Obstetric Complications*,
DOI 10.1007/978-3-319-54410-6_3

Emergency Department Management

Diagnosis

HG is a clinical diagnosis. Emergency department (ED) evaluation begins with a thorough history and physical exam in conjunction with basic laboratory work. The hallmark symptoms of HG are excessive or unrelenting nausea and severe vomiting associated with [7]:

1. Weight loss of greater than 5% prepregnancy weight.
2. Signs of dehydration including orthostatic hypotension, elevated BUN, elevated hematocrit, decreased urine output, and syncope.
3. Presence of ketones in the urine.
4. Electrolyte disturbance including hyponatremia, hypochloremia, and hypokalemia [8].

Relevant predisposing risk factors for HG include female fetus, multiple pregnancy, prior personal or family history of HG, and molar pregnancy [9, 10]. Additional elements in the history that may point toward HG include a report of hypersensitivity to smells, hypersalivation, and symptoms suggestive of dehydration such as feeling lightheaded, dizziness, or syncope. Suggested laboratory tests include urinalysis, basic metabolic panel, and liver function tests (Table 3.1).

If no prior prenatal care has been received, an ultrasound should also be obtained to ensure an intrauterine pregnancy is present and there is no evidence of trophoblastic disease. Transient depressed thyroid stimulating hormone occurs in up to 60% of patients with HG [11]. However, these patients are clinically euthyroid and do not require further treatment to correct thyroid levels [12]. Routine testing of thyroid function in the ED is not necessary in patients with HG.

Table 3.1 Recommended laboratory testing for evaluation of hyperemesis gravidarum

Test	Abnormalities seen in hyperemesis gravidarum
Urinalysis	Elevated urine specific gravity (>1.020) Presence of ketones
Basic metabolic panel	Electrolyte disturbances (hyponatremia, hypochloremia, hypokalemia) Acidosis Elevated BUN Evidence of acute kidney injury
Liver function tests	Elevated AST/ALT and total bilirubin may occur in up to 50% of HG patients

Treatment

A stepwise approach to the treatment of mild nausea and vomiting of pregnancy and HG in the emergency department is recommended (Table 3.2). Early recognition and treatment of nausea and vomiting in pregnancy is essential to minimize the impact of symptoms and prevent further disease progression. The first step is to restore normal volume status. Oral rehydration may be sufficient for more mild symptoms if tolerated by the patient. In cases of moderate to severe dehydration or inability to tolerate oral intake, intravenous fluids are required. Other therapies to consider for supportive care include vitamin repletion, specifically thiamine and folate, along with dextrose if prolonged symptoms. Lifestyle modifications and the use of alternative therapies can be suggested. Lifestyle changes commonly recommended include dietary changes and avoidance of triggers. Patients should be encouraged to take small continuous sips of neutral liquids (i.e., ginger ale) or electrolyte sports drinks. Eating small, frequent bland snacks (i.e., saltine crackers) to avoid an empty stomach may also decrease nausea [13]. A non-pharmacological alternative therapy that is considered safe in pregnancy is ginger supplements. Several small studies have shown benefit of ginger supplements in the reduction of nausea and vomiting in pregnancy when compared to placebo [14, 15]. Ginger supplements can be administered as 250 mg four times daily [16].

For patients with symptoms refractory to lifestyle and dietary modifications who require pharmacological antiemetic therapy, pyridoxine (vitamin B6) alone or pyridoxine with doxylamine is considered first-line therapy and recommended by the American College of Obstetricians and Gynecologists (ACOG) [17].

Historically, pyridoxine and doxylamine was sold in the USA as Bendectin from 1956 to 1983. Despite claims in the 1970s and 1980s of possible teratogenic effects of Bendectin, the Food and Drug Administration (FDA) found no link between Bendectin and human birth defects [18, 19]. Subsequently, the voluntary removal of Bendectin from the US market did not correlate with a reduction in birth defect reports, and the hospitalization rate for women with hyperemesis gravidarum doubled [20–22].

The use of pyridoxine with doxylamine has been shown to be safe and effective in the treatment of nausea and vomiting in pregnancy in the meta-analysis of multiple cohort and case-control studies [23]. A 2015 matched, controlled cohort study found improved nausea control with pyridoxine with doxylamine therapy in comparison to pyridoxine therapy alone. This difference was most evident in patients with moderate to severe symptoms [24]. Pyridoxine with doxylamine has been available commercially in the USA as a delayed-release combination 10 mg/10 mg tablet under the brand name Diclegis® since 2013 and remains the only FDA-approved medication for the treatment of nausea and vomiting in pregnancy with an FDA pregnancy category A rating [25] (Table 3.3). For patients discharged from the

Table 3.2 Recommended treatment algorithm for nausea and vomiting in pregnancy

Step in therapy	Treatment option	Clinical considerations
1. Supportive care	• Restoration of normal volume status with oral (if tolerated) or IV fluids (D5 ½ normal saline) • Add 20 mEq KCL if hypokalemic • Vitamin repletion • A multivitamin containing folate	Avoid rapid correction of hyponatremia Consider thiamine repletion, especially prior to dextrose administration if prolonged symptoms or concern for Wernicke's encephalopathy
2. Antiemetic therapy: first line	• Diclegis®, pyridoxine 10 mg + doxylamine 10 mg (two pills taken at bedtime) • Pyridoxine 25 mg every 6 h + doxylamine 12.5 mg every 6 h	Diclegis®: pregnancy category A Onset of action 5–7 h, oral dose only, ideal for home use
3. Antiemetic therapy: second line, for moderate to severe vomiting	• H1 antagonists Diphenhydramine 25 mg every 6 h or dimenhydrinate 50 mg every 6 h	Diphenhydramine: pregnancy category B Side effects: sedation, dry mouth, urinary retention
	• Dopamine antagonists: Metoclopramide 10 mg	Metoclopramide: pregnancy category B Side effects: sedation, tardive dyskinesia, acute dystonic reaction
4. Antiemetic therapy: alternate second line, for refractory symptoms	• Selective serotonin antagonists Ondansetron 4 mg every 8 h, maximum 16 mg IV	Ondansetron: pregnancy category B, high efficacy in studies Recommend EKG and electrolyte monitoring with IV use Side effects: maternal QT prolongation in IV formulation, may cause fetal cardiac septum malformation
	• Phenothiazines Prochlorperazine 10 mg every 6 h or promethazine 25 mg every 4 h	Promethazine: pregnancy category C, may be administered rectally Prochlorperazine: less well studied
	• Steroids Methylprednisolone 40 mg daily, after 10 weeks' gestation, limit 3-day therapy	Steroids: may cause fetal oral clefts, low birth weight, last resort therapy, routine use not recommended
5. Adjunctive treatments	• Dietary changes Eat bland foods, small frequent meals, avoid having an empty stomach	No reported adverse effects
	• Avoidance of triggers Especially olfactory triggers	No reported adverse effects
	• Supplements Ginger 250 mg supplements four times daily	Avoid supplements with multiple active ingredients with unknown safety profiles

ED with nausea and vomiting in pregnancy, Diclegis® remains the recommended prescription therapy due to its delayed-release formulation. Diclegis® should be used daily rather than on an as-needed basis. Diclegis® is prescribed with the initial dose of two tablets at bedtime to address morning symptoms. If symptoms persist in the afternoon, an additional tablet may be taken in the morning, up to four tablets per

Table 3.3 FDA drug risk classification in pregnancy[a]

Category	Description
A	Controlled studies in humans show no risk to the fetus
B	Animal studies show no risk to the fetus, no controlled studies in humans
C	No controlled studies in animals or humans
D	Evidence of human risk to the fetus exists; however, benefits may outweigh risks
X	Controlled studies demonstrate fetal abnormalities. Risk outweighs any possible benefit

[a]As of 2014 the FDA is changing drug labeling regarding use during pregnancy or lactation and phasing out the letter categories [42]

day [26]. Diclegis® is expensive for some patients and not covered by all insurances. As an alternative, clinicians may prescribe doxylamine 12.5 mg by mouth every 6 h and pyridoxine 25 mg by mouth every 6 h. However, over-the-counter immediate-release doxylamine has not been shown to have similar therapeutic efficacy, exhibits higher sedative effects than the delayed-release formulation, and may contain other active ingredients that have not been studied for safety in pregnancy [25].

Pyridoxine with doxylamine is not approved for IV administration or for the treatment of HG. Other antiemetic therapies should be considered in patients with persistent nausea and vomiting or HG. These medications include H1 antagonists, selective serotonin inhibitors, and dopamine antagonists (Table 3.2). These medications have limited fetal safety data and are used off-label in the treatment of nausea and vomiting in pregnancy. Maternal benefit versus fetal safety should be weighed when considering these options.

H1 antagonists used in pregnancy include diphenhydramine, dimenhydrinate, and meclizine. These medications hold an FDA pregnancy category B rating; however, there are no well-controlled studies of fetal safety with these medications [28]. These medications may cause maternal drowsiness.

Metoclopramide is a dopamine receptor antagonist classified as FDA pregnancy category B and is used off-label for HG. A large retrospective cohort study evaluating for congenital malformations, perinatal death, low birth weight, and low Apgar scores found no adverse pregnancy or fetal outcomes associated with metoclopramide use in first trimester of pregnancy [27]. Metoclopramide may cause drowsiness and dizziness and comes with risk of acute dystonic reactions and tardive dyskinesia. Risk of serotonin syndrome with concomitant use of antidepressants should be considered. Promethazine and prochlorperazine are additional dopamine receptor antagonists to be considered as third-line agents, as promethazine is a category C medication and limited safety data exists for prochlorperazine [28]. Promethazine may be administered rectally if the patient is unable to tolerate any oral medications.

Ondansetron is a 5-HT3 receptor antagonist that is designated by the FDA as pregnancy category B. Several studies have shown it to be as effective and perhaps more effective compared to other commonly used antiemetics including pyridoxine in the treatment of nausea and vomiting in pregnancy [29, 30]. One study comparing ondansetron to metoclopramide showed not only similar efficacy but also less adverse effects including decreased drowsiness with use of ondansetron [31].

Several small studies as well as two large retrospective cohort studies have reported conflicting results as to the safety of ondansetron in pregnancy. A large retrospective cohort study by Pasternak et al. included 608,385 pregnant patients in Denmark. This study compared the risk of several adverse fetal outcomes including spontaneous abortion, stillbirth, any major birth defect, preterm delivery, and low birth weight between pregnant women exposed to ondansetron and women not exposed. They found that exposure to ondansetron was not associated with a significantly increased risk of any of the adverse fetal outcomes studied [32]. Another large cohort study by Danielsson et al. was performed using data from the Swedish Medical Birth Register. The authors found no statistically significant increased risk for major fetal malformation. This study did, however, show a statistically significant increased risk of cardiovascular defects, specifically cardiac septum defects among neonates exposed to maternal ondansetron use (OR = 1.62, 95% CI 1.04–2.14, and RR 2.05, 95% CI 1.19–3.28, respectively) [33]. The analysis by Danielsson et al., however, was less rigorous (adjusted for fewer confounders, importantly maternal medical history), as compared to the study by Pasternak et al.

Two systematic reviews of current literature on ondansetron use in pregnancy were conducted in the past year. One review performed by Siminerio et al. concluded that current data does not support avoiding ondansetron in the treatment of pregnant women based on "the principle of absence of harm to date and presence of efficacy." The authors concluded that maternal benefit outweighs potential risk [34]. A separate systematic review recommends reserving ondansetron for women whose symptoms are not adequately controlled by other treatments given reports of a small increase in the incidence of neonate cardiac abnormalities with maternal ondansetron use [35]. Maternal risks with intravenous ondansetron use include QT prolongation and risk of torsades de pointes. Intravenous doses should be limited to 16 mg and require EKG and electrolyte monitoring per FDA recommendations [36].

The use of steroids for the treatment of HG remains controversial. Studies have yielded conflicting results regarding fetal outcomes of prenatal maternal systemic steroid use. Steroids have been linked to low birth weight and low head circumference as well as mixed reports of an increase in cleft lip and cleft palate [37–39]. A systematic review and meta-analysis on the utility of steroid use in the treatment of HG concluded that there was insufficient evidence to support its use [18]. ACOG states that methylprednisolone may be of benefit in refractory cases of HG; however, given its risk profile, it should be a last resort after 10 weeks' gestation [20]. The authors do not recommend the routine use of steroids in HG in the emergency department. The decision to use steroids as a last resort should be made in consultation with an obstetrician.

Disposition

The majority of patients presenting to the emergency department with nausea and vomiting in pregnancy can be safely discharged at home. Admission to the hospital is reserved for persistent/severe nausea and vomiting, severe dehydration, or lab

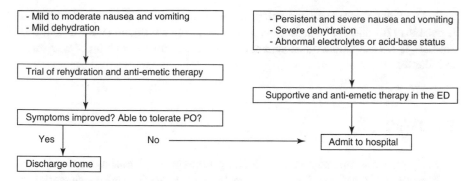

Fig. 3.1 Disposition algorithm for nausea and vomiting in pregnancy

abnormalities including electrolyte or acid-base derangements that require intravenous correction (Fig. 3.1). For patients discharged from the emergency department, close obstetrics follow-up, dietary counseling, and prescription of pyridoxine with doxylamine as first-line preventive therapy are indicated.

Complications

Although rare, there are several important potential maternal complications associated with HG. These include, but are not limited to, Wernicke's encephalopathy (WE), osmotic demyelination syndrome from overly rapid correction of hyponatremia, esophageal rupture, Mallory-Weiss tears, pneumomediastinum from forceful vomiting, and acute tubular necrosis [23]. As of 2010 there were only 49 cases reported in the literature of WE in pregnancy [40]. Despite the rarity of this complication, WE can lead to devastating and persistent neurologic sequelae with complete remission observed in only 14 of the reported cases [41]. Thiamine repletion before dextrose infusion is therefore a critical intervention in patients that have had prolonged vomiting and concern for nutritional compromise.

Summary

Nausea and vomiting affects up to 80% of pregnancies and can have significant negative impact on the patient's quality of life. Prompt treatment is essential to preventing further progression of symptoms. Initial evaluation of the pregnant patient with nausea and vomiting in the ED should focus on detecting more severe disease including dehydration, electrolyte imbalances, and hyperemesis gravidarum. In addition to supportive care with fluid and volume repletion, first-line pharmacologic therapy should consist of pyridoxine with doxylamine. Patients with persistent symptoms can be managed with additional antiemetic agents including diphenhydramine, metoclopramide, and ondansetron. Hospital admission is necessary for cases of refractory vomiting requiring continued IV fluids and antiemetics, failed outpatient management of symptoms, and severe fluid or electrolyte imbalance.

Key Points

- Early prevention of nausea and vomiting in pregnancy consists of dietary and lifestyle modifications: bland diet, small frequent meals, and consideration of ginger supplements.
- Pyridoxine with doxylamine remains the first-line pharmacotherapy for outpatient treatment of nausea and vomiting in pregnancy and may prevent repeat ED visits and the development of severe symptoms.
- Diphenhydramine, metoclopramide, and ondansetron used off-label use are second-line agents to consider in refractory cases.
- Recommended ED laboratory evaluation includes urinalysis, basic metabolic panel, and liver function tests to assess for electrolyte abnormalities and severity of dehydration.
- Consider thiamine, folate, and dextrose in cases of severe or prolonged symptoms.

References

1. Einarson TR, Piwko C, Koren G. Prevalence of nausea and vomiting of pregnancy in the USA: a meta analysis. J Popul Ther Clin Pharmacol. 2013;20(2):e163–70.
2. Piwko C, Koren G, Babashov V, Vicente C, Einarson TR. Economic Burden of nausea and vomiting of pregnancy in the USA. J Popul Ther Clin Pharmacol. 2013;20(2):e149–60. Epub 2013 Jul 10
3. Sheehan P. Hyperemesis gravidarum – assessment and management. Aust Fam Physician. 2007;36(9):698–701.
4. Boelig RC, Barton SJ, Saccone G, Kelly AJ, Edwards SJ, Berghella V. Interventions for treating hyperemesis gravidarum. Cochrane Database Syst Rev. 2016;(5). Art. No.: CD010607.
5. Eliakim R, Abulafiaz O, Shere DM. Hyperemesis gravidarum: a current review. Am J Perinatol. 2000;17(4):207–18.
6. Body C, Christie J. Gastrointestinal disease in pregnancy. Gastroenterol Clin North Am. 2016;45:267–83.
7. World Health Organization. International classification of diseases: 10. Version: 2010. 2012. http://tinyurl.com/ctcuekp. Accessed 29 June 2016.
8. Summers A. Emergency management of hyperemesis gravidarum. Emerg Nurse. 2012;20(4):24–8.
9. Kuscu NK, Koyuncu F. Hyperemesis gravidarum: current concepts and management. Postgrad Med J. 2002;78(916):76–9.
10. Zhang Y, Cantor RM, MacGibbon K, Romero R, Goodwin TM, Mullin PM, Feizo MS. Familial aggregation of hyperemesis gravidarum. Am J Obstet Gynecol. 2011;204(3):230.e1–7.

11. Schiff MA, Reed SD, Daling JR. The sex ratio of pregnancies complicated by hospitalisation for hyperemesis gravidarum. BJOG. 2004;111:27–30.
12. Tan JYL, Loh KC, Yeo GSH, Chee YC. Transient hyperthyroidism of hyperemesis gravidarum. BJOG. 2002;109:683–8.
13. Ismail SK, Kenny L. Review on hyperemesis gravidarum. Clin Gastroenterol. 2007;21(5):755–69.
14. Vutyavanich T, Kraisarin T, Ruangsri R. Ginger for nausea and vomiting in pregnancy: randomised, double masked, placebo controlled trial. Obstet Gynecol. 2001;97:577–82.
15. Fischer-Rasmussen W, Kiaer SK, Dahl C, Asping U. Ginger treatment of hyperemesis gravidarum. Eur J Obstet Gynecol Reprod Biol. 1991;38(1):19–24.
16. Borrelli F, Capasso R, Aviello G, et al. Effectiveness and safety of ginger in the treatment of pregnancy-induced nausea and vomiting. Obstet Gynecol. 2005;105(4):849–56.
17. American College of Obstetricians and Gynecologists Practice Bulletin. Number 153. 2015. http://dx.doi.org/10.1097/AOG.0000000000001048. Accessed 29 June 2016.
18. Grooten IJ, et al. A systematic review and meta-analysis of the utility of corticosteroids in the treatment of hyperemesis gravidarum. Nutr Metab Insights. 2015;8(S1):23–32.
19. Duchesnay Inc. Bendectin history. 2013. http://www.bendectin.com/en. Accessed 29 June 2016
20. American College of Obstetrics and Gynecology. Practice Bulletin No 153.
21. Kutcher JS, Engle A, Firth J, Lamm SH. Bendectin and birth defects. II: ecological analyses. Birth Defects Res A Clin Mol Teratol. 2003;67(2):88–97.
22. McKeigue PM, Lamm SH, Linn S, Kutcher JS. Bendectin and birth defects: I. A meta-analysis of the epidemiologic studies. Teratology. 1994;50(1):27–37.
23. Goodwin T. Murphy hyperemesis gravidarum. Obstet Gynecol Clin. 2008;35(3):401–17.
24. Pope E, Maltepe C, Koren G. Comparing pyridoxine and doxylamine succinate-pyridoxine HCl for nausea and vomiting of pregnancy: a matched, controlled cohort study. J Clin Pharmacol. 2015;55(7):809–14.
25. Madjunkova S, Maltepe C, Koren G. The delayed-release combination of doxylamine and pyridoxine (Diclegis/Diclectin) for the treatment of nausea and vomiting of pregnancy. Paediatr Drugs. 2014;16(3):199–211.
26. Tobin S. Management of nausea and vomiting of pregnancy after discharge from the Emergency Department. Emerg Med News Duchesnay Suppl. 2016.
27. Matok I, Gorodischer R, Koren G, Sheiner E, Wiznitzer A, Levy A. The safety of metoclopramide use in the first trimester of pregnancy. N Engl J Med. 2009;360(24):2528–35.
28. Magee LA, Mazzotta P, Koren G. Evidence-based view of safety and effectiveness of pharmacologic therapy for nausea and vomiting of pregnancy (NVP). Am J Obstet Gynecol. 2002;186(5 Suppl Understanding):S256–61. 37
29. Mayhall EA, Gray R, Lopes V, Matteson KA. Comparison of antiemetics for nausea and vomiting of pregnancy in an emergency department setting. Am J Emerg Med. 2015;33:882–6.
30. Oliveira LG, Capp SM, You WB, Riffenburgh RH, Carstairs SD. Ondansetron compared with doxylamine and pyridoxine for treatment of nausea in pregnancy. Obstet Gynecol. 2014;124:735–42.
31. Abas MN, Tan PC, Azmi N, Omar SZ. Ondansetron compared with metoclopramide for hyperemesis gravidarum: a randomized controlled trial. Obstet Gynecol. 2014;123:1272–9.
32. Pasternak B, Svanström H, Hvild A. Ondansetron in pregnancy and risk of adverse fetal outcomes. N Engl J Med. 2013;368:814–23. Erratum in N Engl J Med 2013;368:2146
33. Danielsson B, Wikner BN, Källén B. Use of ondansetron during pregnancy and congenital malformations in the infant. Reprod Toxicol. 2014;50:134–7.
34. Siminerio L, Bodnar L, Venkataramanan R, Caritis S. Ondansetron use in pregnancy. Obstet Gynecol. 2016;127:873–7.
35. Carstairs S. Ondansetron use in pregnancy and birth defects. Obstet Gynecol. 2016;127:878–83.
36. Freedman SB, Uleryk E, Rumantir M, et al. Ondansetron and the risk of cardiac arrhythmias: a systematic review and postmarketing analysis. Ann Emerg Med. 2014;64(1):19–25. e16

37. Carmichael SL, Shaw GM, Ma C, et al. Maternal corticosteroid use and orofacial clefts. Am J Obstet Gynecol. 2007;197(6):585. e581–7. Discussion 683–684, e581–587.
38. Skuladottir H, Wilcox AJ, Ma C, et al. Corticosteroid use and risk of orofacial clefts. Birth Defects Res A Clin Mol Teratol. 2014;100(6):499–506.
39. Painter RC, Roseboom TJ, de Rooij SR. Long-term effects of prenatal stress and glucocorticoid exposure. Birth Defects Res C Embryo Today. 2012;96(4):315–24.
40. Togay-Isikay C, Yigit A, Mutluer N. Wernicke's encephalopathy due to hyperemesis gravidarum: an under-recognised condition. Aust N Z J Obstet.Gynaecol. 2001;41:453–6.
41. Chiossi G, Neri I, Cavazzuti M, Basso G, Facchinetti F. Hyperemesis gravidarum complicated by Wernicke encephalopathy: background, case report, and review of the literature. Obstet Gynecol Surv. 2006;61(4):255–68.
42. Food and Drug Administration. Content and format of labeling for human prescription drug and biological products; requirements for pregnancy and lactation labeling. 2014. https://federalregister.gov/a/2014-28241.

Chapter 4
Hypertensive Disorders of Pregnancy

Whitney Sherman, Edward Descallar, and Joelle Borhart

Introduction

Hypertension is the most common medical disorder of pregnancy, complicating up to 10% of gestations [1]. Preeclampsia is a leading cause of maternal and perinatal morbidity and mortality and the incidence in increasing [2]. It is estimated that for every preeclampsia-related death, 50–100 women experience a "near-miss" event resulting in significant health risk and morbidity [3, 4]. Many women in the second or third trimester of pregnancy present to the emergency department (ED) for a variety of reasons, and emergency physicians are in a unique position to identify and treat patients with a hypertensive disorder of pregnancy before serious complications occur.

Classification of Hypertensive Disorders of Pregnancy

In 2013, the American College of Obstetricians and Gynecologists' (ACOG) Task Force on Hypertension in Pregnancy released updated evidence-based guidelines for the diagnosis and management of hypertensive disorders of pregnancy [5]. The task force divides hypertension in pregnancy into four categories: (1) preeclampsia/eclampsia, (2) chronic hypertension, (3) chronic hypertension with superimposed preeclampsia, and (4) gestational hypertension (Table 4.1). Hypertension in pregnancy is defined as either a systolic blood pressure of 140 mmHg or greater or a diastolic blood pressure of 90 mmHg or greater. Blood pressure should be elevated on at least two separate occasions more than 4 h apart before the diagnosis of

W. Sherman, M.D. • E. Descallar, M.D. • J. Borhart, M.D. (✉)
Department of Emergency Medicine, MedStar Georgetown University Hospital and MedStar Washington Hospital Center, 3800 Reservoir Road NW, Washington, DC 20007, USA
e-mail: wredline@gmail.com; descallare@gmail.com; joelle.borhart@gmail.com

© Springer International Publishing AG 2017
J. Borhart (ed.), *Emergency Department Management of Obstetric Complications*,
DOI 10.1007/978-3-319-54410-6_4

Table 4.1 Definitions of the Hypertensive Disorders of Pregnancy

Hypertensive disorder of pregnancy	Diagnostic criteria
Preeclampsia	New-onset hypertension (blood pressure >140 mmHg systolic and/or >90 mmHg diastolic) after 20 weeks and proteinuria Or in the absence of proteinuria: New-onset hypertension after 20 weeks and signs/symptoms of end-organ damage (Box 4.1)
Eclampsia	New-onset seizures in woman with preeclampsia
Chronic hypertension	Hypertension that predates pregnancy or is diagnosed before 20 weeks
Chronic hypertension with superimposed preeclampsia	Patients with chronic hypertension that develop preeclampsia
Gestational hypertension	New-onset hypertension after 20 weeks without proteinuria or signs/symptoms of preeclampsia

Adapted from American College of Obstetricians and Gynecologists, Task Force on Hypertension in Pregnancy. Hypertension in pregnancy. Report of the American College of Obstetricians and Gynecologists' task force on hypertension in pregnancy Obstet Gynecol. 2013;122:1122–1131

hypertension is made. However, even an isolated elevated blood pressure reading is concerning, especially if the blood pressure is greater than 160 mmHg systolic and/or 110 mmHg diastolic.

Preeclampsia has traditionally been defined as new onset of hypertension plus proteinuria after 20 weeks of gestation. Proteinuria is defined as excretion of 300 mg or more of protein in a 24-h urine collection or a random protein/creatinine ratio of at least 0.3 mg/dL. Urine dipstick is discouraged to diagnose proteinuria unless other methods are unavailable, in which case a measurement of at least 1+ must be obtained.

Importantly, the task force has eliminated the requirement of proteinuria to make the diagnosis of preeclampsia. In the absence of proteinuria, preeclampsia can be diagnosed in the setting of hypertension after 20 weeks of gestation plus signs or symptoms of end-organ damage, also called "severe features" (Box 4.1). Eclampsia is defined as new-onset grand mal seizures in women with preeclampsia and can occur before, during, or after labor.

HELLP syndrome is an acronym for hemolysis (H), elevated liver enzymes (EL), and low platelets (LP). Many authors consider HELLP syndrome to be a complication of preeclampsia and eclampsia, though some feel HELLP syndrome to be separate entity [6]. Hypertension may be mild or absent in patients with HELLP syndrome (Box 4.2).

Chronic hypertension is hypertension that predates pregnancy or is diagnosed before 20 weeks of gestation. Patients with chronic hypertension may develop preeclampsia, and this is referred to as superimposed preeclampsia. Gestational hypertension is hypertension that occurs after 20 weeks without proteinuria or other signs/symptoms of preeclampsia. However, gestational hypertension is not a benign diagnosis—between 15 and 25% of women with gestational hypertension will develop preeclampsia [7].

Box 4.1 Severe features of preeclampsia

- Systolic blood pressure >160 mmHg or diastolic >110 mmHg
- Thrombocytopenia (platelet count <100,000/μL)
- Impaired liver function (twice normal)
- Severe persistent right upper quadrant or epigastric pain unresponsive to medication
- Renal insufficiency (creatinine >1.1 mg/dL or doubling of creatinine in absence of other renal disease)
- Pulmonary edema
- New-onset cerebral or visual disturbances

Adapted from American College of Obstetricians and Gynecologists, Task Force on Hypertension in Pregnancy. Hypertension in pregnancy. Report of the American College of Obstetricians and Gynecologists' task force on hypertension in pregnancy. Obstet Gynecol. 2013;122:1122–11

Box 4.2 Diagnosis of HELLP syndrome

- Evidence of hemolysis:
  - Schistocytes on peripheral smear
  - Lactate dehydrogenase >600 IU/L
  - Total bilirubin 1.2 mg/dL
- Elevated aspartate aminotransferase (>70 IU/L)
- Thrombocytopenia (platelets <100,000/μL)

Adapted from Olsen-Chen C, Seligman NS. Hypertensive emergencies in pregnancy. Crit Care Clin. 2016;32:29–41

Pathophysiology

The concept of preeclampsia/eclampsia has been recognized since ancient times [8], yet the exact mechanisms leading to the disorder still remain unclear. Some women may be genetically predisposed to developing the disease. Recent research suggests that poor placentation can lead to placental hypoxia and insufficiency causing a complex cascade of endothelial dysfunction leading to many of the clinical features observed in preeclampsia [9, 10].

Emergency Department Management

Evaluation

Pregnant patients that are greater than 20 weeks of gestational age presenting to the emergency department (ED) for any reason and are noted to be hypertensive must be evaluated for signs and symptoms of end-organ damage to rule out preeclampsia. Patients should be asked about the presence of headache, visual changes, abdominal pain (specifically right upper quadrant or epigastric pain), chest pain, and shortness of breath. As many women with preeclampsia may have no symptoms [11], laboratory tests are necessary. Minimum laboratory test includes complete blood count to evaluate for thrombocytopenia, complete metabolic panel to assess creatinine level and liver enzymes, and urinalysis or urine protein/creatinine ratio to evaluate for proteinuria. Additional tests can include lactate dehydrogenase to evaluate for hemolysis if there is concern for HELLP syndrome, coagulation studies, and baseline magnesium level. Serum uric acid may also be ordered as elevated levels have been associated with adverse maternal and fetal outcomes and may help identify women with gestational hypertension who will progress to preeclampsia [12, 13].

Treatment

Delivery is the definitive treatment for preeclampsia, eclampsia, and HELLP syndrome. Timing of delivery is dependent on maternal condition and gestational age of the fetus. Emergency department treatment of the preeclamptic or eclamptic patient includes controlling blood pressure, initiating seizure prophylaxis, treating seizures if they occur, and obtaining emergent obstetric consultation.

Control of Blood Pressure

Pregnant women with blood pressure >160 mmHg systolic or >110 mmHg diastolic require antihypertensive therapy to reduce the risk of stroke and other maternal complications. The goal is to stabilize blood pressure around 140/90 mmHg, not to normalize blood pressure [14]. Sudden drops in blood pressure should be avoided so as not to cause additional complications such as fetal distress.

There is no consensus on an ideal agent for treating blood pressure in preeclampsia [15]. Clinicians should select a drug based on maternal characteristics/contraindications and their own familiarity and experience with a medication. All antihypertensive drugs used in pregnancy cross the placenta, so possible effects on the fetus should also be taken into consideration. The most commonly used agents are labetalol, hydralazine, and nifedipine. All three drugs may be considered first-line therapy. Suggested dosing regimens and drug characteristics are outlined in Tables 4.2 and 4.3, respectively. Magnesium is not recommended as an antihypertensive agent [14].

Seizure Prophylaxis and Treatment

For women with preeclampsia with severe features, magnesium sulfate should be given as prophylaxis against eclampsia [5]. The suggested dose for seizure prophylaxis is 4 g IV over 5 min, followed by 1 g/h infusion. Treatment with magnesium sulfate has been shown to reduce the risk of eclampsia by half [16].

Table 4.2 Initial approach for management of severe antepartum, intrapartum, or postpartum hypertension

Labetalol	Hydralazine	Nifedipine
If BP remains >160 mmHg systolic or >110 diastolic for more than 15 min:		
Give 20 mg IV over 2 min Repeat BP in 10 min	Give 5–10 mg IV over 2 min Repeat BP in 20 min	Give 10 mg orally Repeat BP in 20 min
If BP remains >160 mmHg systolic or >110 diastolic:		
Give 40 mg IV over 2 min Repeat BP in 10 min	Give 10 mg IV over 2 min Repeat BP in 20 min	Give 20 mg orally Repeat BP in 20 min
If BP remains >160 mmHg systolic or >110 diastolic:		
Give 80 mg IV over 2 min Repeat BP in 10 min	Give labetalol 20 mg IV over 2 min Repeat BP in 10 min	Give 20 mg orally Repeat BP in 20 min
If BP remains >160 mmHg systolic or >110 diastolic:		
Give hydralazine 10 mg IV over 2 min Repeat BP in 20 min	Give labetalol 40 mg IV over 2 min Repeat BP in 10 min	Give labetalol 40 mg IV over 2 min Repeat BP in 10 min
If BP remains >160 mmHg systolic or >110 diastolic:		
Obtain emergent consultation from obstetrics, maternal-fetal medicine, or critical care subspecialists and treat as recommended		
Once target BP reached, repeat BP every 10 min for 1 h, then every 15 min for 1 h, then every 30 min for 1 h, then every hour for 4 h		

Abbreviations: BP blood pressure, *IV* intravenous. Adapted from American College of Obstetricians and Gynecologists. Committee Opinion No 623: emergent therapy for acute-onset, severe hypertension during pregnancy and the postpartum period. Obstet Gynecol. 2015;125:521–525

Table 4.3 Characteristics of antihypertensive drugs commonly used for severe hypertension in pregnancy

Drug	Mechanism	Contraindications/cautions
Labetalol	Nonselective beta-blocker, some alpha-blocking activity	Avoid in women with asthma, heart disease, congestive heart failure May cause neonatal bradycardia and hypoglycemia
Hydralazine	Direct vasodilator, relaxes arteriolar smooth muscle	May cause maternal hypotension, tachycardia, headache, flushing, nausea/vomiting, palpitations
Nifedipine	Calcium channel blocker	May cause maternal tachycardia, flushing, palpitations, headache

Adapted from Olsen-Chen C, Seligman NS. Hypertensive emergencies in pregnancy. Crit Care Clin. 2016;32:29–41

If seizures develop, magnesium sulfate is still the drug of choice and has been shown to be superior to diazepam, phenytoin, and lytic cocktail in reducing maternal death and further seizures [17–19]. If magnesium has not been started yet, give 4 g IV over 5 min, then 1 g/h infusion. If the patient is already receiving magnesium and seizes, give an additional 2–4 g IV over 5 min and increase the infusion to 2 g/h [20]. Eclamptic seizures are generally short in duration (<1 min) [21]. Cerebral imaging should be considered for patients with prolonged or repeated seizures and for patients with a focal neurologic deficit to rule out possible intracranial hemorrhage or other neurologic complication.

Patients receiving magnesium should be closely monitored for signs of magnesium toxicity. Symptoms of magnesium toxicity include loss of deep tendon reflexes, respiratory depression, somnolence, and cardiac arrest. If magnesium toxicity is suspected, the infusion should be stopped immediately and 10 mL of 10% calcium gluconate can be administered [22]. There is theoretical concern that treatment with both nifedipine and magnesium sulfate could result in increased risk of magnesium-related maternal side effects such neuromuscular blockade and severe hypotension, but this has not been shown to be the case [23].

Disposition

The progression of preeclampsia is unpredictable and can be rapid; therefore, hospital admission to an obstetrics unit is usually indicated. The emergency physician must decide if the current facility has the capacity and capability to provide the level of maternal-fetal-neonatal care needed or if the patient would benefit from transfer to a higher level of care. Transfer of patients to a facility with sufficient obstetric and neonatal resources has been shown to reduce maternal, fetal, and neonatal morbidity and mortality [24]. Since the definitive treatment of preeclampsia and eclampsia is delivery, the decision of when and where to transfer is often based on gestational age and the need for obstetric and neonatal specialists [25]. Neonatal mortality is significantly lower if preterm babies are delivered at highly specialized hospitals rather than being transported there after birth [26, 27]. For this reason, every effort should be made to transfer a pregnant patient with preeclampsia/eclampsia to a tertiary care facility prior to delivery, especially if she is far from term.

The Emergency Medical Treatment and Active Labor Act (EMTALA) imposes specific obligations on healthcare providers to perform a medical screening examination and to provide stabilizing treatment to any patient with an emergency medical condition [28]. In pregnant women, this includes both the mother and fetus. According to EMTALA, a woman in labor is considered unstable until both the baby and the placenta have been delivered. However, a patient in labor may still be transferred if there is felt to be adequate time before delivery or if the benefits of transfer outweigh the risks. Several steps must be taken before transfer can take place: (1) assessment of fetal viability, gestational age, and well-being; (2) stabilizing treatment with control of blood pressure and convulsions and seizure prophylaxis with a loading dose of magnesium sulfate if appropriate; (3) maternal laboratory assessment (complete blood count and platelet count, liver enzymes, creatinine, urine protein); (4) fetal monitoring if available; (5) consultation of obstetric/perinatal team; and (6) transmission of all records for review [27].

Special Considerations

Postpartum Preeclampsia

The majority of hypertensive emergencies associated with pregnancy occur antepartum or within the first 48 h after delivery [29]. Eclampsia that occurs greater than 48 h after delivery is known as late postpartum eclampsia (LPPE) [30]. The incidence of LPPE appears to be increasing and now represents about 13–16% of all cases of eclampsia [31–34]. Blood pressure has been shown to rise over the first week after delivery and peaks on postpartum days 3–6 [35, 36]. This is likely due to physiologic fluid mobilization and volume expansion. The use of medications such as nonsteroidal anti-inflammatory pills, ergot derivatives, and decongestants may also contribute to postpartum hypertension [36, 37].

Preeclampsia and eclampsia may occur up to 6 weeks postpartum. Women who develop postpartum preeclampsia and eclampsia may have had no evidence of the disease during their pregnancy [38]. Many women in the postpartum period may present to the emergency department for evaluation instead of being seen by their obstetric provider. Early treatment of preeclampsia, eclampsia, and HELLP syndrome in the postpartum patient hinges on whether the clinician recognizes late presentations of these disorders. The criteria for diagnosing postpartum preeclampsia, eclampsia, and HELLP syndrome are the same as in the antepartum period.

In the postpartum period, headache is the most common presenting symptom of preeclampsia [38]. It should be noted that headache could also herald other potentially serious conditions. An estimated 10–11% of postpartum patients with headache have critical conditions such as intracranial bleed, stroke, mass, or cerebral venous sinus thrombosis [39]. Patients with postpartum preeclampsia may also present with abdominal pain, chest pain, shortness of breath, visual changes, or increased swelling, similar to antepartum patients.

Preeclampsia and eclampsia in the postpartum period should be managed the same as antepartum period by controlling blood pressure and initiating magnesium sulfate for seizure prophylaxis/control.

HELLP syndrome may develop first in the postpartum period in up to 30% of cases and should be considered in any patient with abdominal pain, nausea, or vomiting [40]. Management is similar to treatment in the antepartum period and includes magnesium sulfate, blood pressure control, and close monitoring of vital signs and laboratory values [37]. The use of steroids for the treatment of HELLP syndrome is conflicting. Some reports have shown improvement in platelet counts following treatment with steroids. However, a 2010 Cochrane review found no evidence of steroids improving in the clinical outcome [41]. The decision to initiate steroid treatment for HELLP syndrome should be made in consultation with an obstetrician.

Preeclampsia Less Than 20 Weeks of Gestation

As stated, preeclampsia is defined as occurring after 20 weeks of gestation. Very rarely, preeclampsia can occur before 20 weeks, usually in abnormal pregnancies complicated by triploidy, trophoblastic disease, or antiphospholipid antibody syndrome [42, 44–47]. Case reports have been published describing preeclampsia before 20 weeks without these abnormalities, and authors refer to this occurrence as "pure" preeclampsia [48, 49]. This is an extremely unusual phenomenon and not likely to be diagnosed in the emergency department. A much more common scenario—and potential pitfall for emergency physicians—would be a patient presenting with signs/symptoms of preeclampsia who is farther along in her pregnancy than previously thought (incorrect dates) and is in fact greater than 20 weeks of gestation. Emergency physicians should confirm the gestational age of any patient pregnant presenting to the ED with hypertension and ensure the most accurate pregnancy dating method was used.

Chronic Hypertension with Superimposed Preeclampsia

Pregnant patients with chronic hypertension presenting to the ED can be especially challenging for emergency physicians. These patients are at risk for developing superimposed preeclampsia, and clinicians should not be reassured that the patient's blood pressure is "always high." Indeed, 13–40% of patients with chronic hypertension will go on to develop superimposed preeclampsia [50, 51], and these women have higher rates of adverse maternal-fetal outcomes [5]. Superimposed preeclampsia should be suspected when there is a sudden increase in blood pressure that was previously well controlled, new-onset proteinuria or sudden increase in proteinuria, or if any other signs/symptoms of end-organ damage are present. Emergency department management of chronic hypertensive patients with superimposed preeclampsia is the same as patients with preeclampsia.

Summary

Hypertension complicates many pregnancies and is a leading cause of maternal and fetal morbidity and mortality. It is critical that emergency physicians assess the blood pressure of pregnant patients presenting to the ED for any reason and screen for signs/symptoms of end-organ damage. Early identification and appropriate management of the hypertensive disorders of pregnancy can improve outcomes for both mother and baby. Treatment of preeclampsia and eclampsia can begin in the ED and includes blood pressure control and seizure prophylaxis with magnesium sulfate. The definitive treatment of preeclampsia, eclampsia, and HELLP syndrome is delivery. Depending on maternal condition and gestational age, transfer to a tertiary facility may be required.

Key Points

- Pregnant patients that are greater than 20 weeks of gestational age presenting to the ED for any reason and are noted to be hypertensive must be evaluated for signs and symptoms of end-organ damage to rule out preeclampsia.
- Proteinuria is no longer required to make the diagnosis of preeclampsia.
- Labetalol, hydralazine, and nifedipine are all considered first-line treatment for severe hypertension in pregnancy.
- Patients with preeclampsia with severe features require magnesium sulfate therapy for prophylaxis against eclampsia.
- Magnesium sulfate is the drug of choice for treatment of eclamptic seizures.

References

1. Mustafa R, Ahmed S, Gupta A, et al. A comprehensive review of hypertension in pregnancy. J Pregnancy. 2012;2012:1–19.
2. Wallis AB, Saftlas AF, Hsia J, et al. Secular trends in the rates of preeclampsia, eclampsia, and gestational hypertension, United States, 1987-2004. Am J Hypertens. 2008;21:521–6.
3. Kuklina EV, Ayala C, Callaghan WM. Hypertensive disorders and severe obstetric morbidity in the United States. Obstet Gynecol. 2009;113:1299–306.
4. Callaghan WM, Mackay AP, Verg CJ. Identification of severe maternal morbidity during delivery hospitalization, United States, 1991-2003. Am J Obstet Gynecol. 2008;199:133e1–7.
5. American College of Obstetricians and Gynecologists, Task Force on Hypertension in Pregnancy. Hypertension in pregnancy. Report of the American College of Obstetricians and Gynecologists' task force on hypertension in pregnancy. Obstet Gynecol. 2013;122:1122–31.
6. Haram K, Svendsen E, Abildgaard U. The HELLP syndrome: clinical issues and management: a review. BMC Pregnancy Childbirth. 2009;9:8.
7. Saudan P, Brown MA, Buddle ML, et al. Does gestational hypertension become preeclampsia? Br J Obstet Gynaecol. 1998;11:1177–84.
8. Bell MJ. A historical overview of preeclampsia-eclampsia. J Obstet Gynecol Neonatal Nurs. 2010;5:510–8.
9. Redman C. Preeclampsia: a complex and variable disease. Pregnancy Hypertens. 2014;3:241–2.
10. Rosene-Montella K. Common medical problems in pregnancy. In: Goldman-Cecil Medicine 25th edition. Ed. Lee Goldman, Ed. Andrew I Schafer. Philadelphia: Elsevier Saunders, 2016:1610–23.
11. Salam RA, Das JK, Ali A, et al. Diagnosis and management of preeclampsia in community settings in low and middle-income countries. J Family Med Prim Care. 2015;4:501–6.
12. Hawkins TL, Roberts JM, Mangos GJ, et al. Plasma urine acid remains a marker of poor outcome in hypertensive pregnancy: a retrospective cohort study. BJOG. 2012;119:484–92.
13. Bellomo G, Venanzi S, Saronio P, et al. Prognostic significance of serum uric acid in women with gestational hypertension. Hypertension. 2011;58:704–8.
14. American College of Obstetricians and Gynecologists. Committee Opinion No 623: emergent therapy for acute-onset, severe hypertension during pregnancy and the postpartum period. Obstet Gynecol. 2015;125:521–5.
15. Duley L, Meher S, Jones L. Drugs for treatment of very high blood pressure during pregnancy. Cochrane Database Syst Rev. 2013;7:CD001449.
16. Duley L, Gulmezoglu AM, Henderson-Smart DJ, et al. Magnesium sulfate and other anticonvulsants for women with preeclampsia. Cochrane Database Syst Rev. 2010;11:CD000025.

17. Duley L, Henderson-Smart DJ, Walker GJ, et al. Magnesium sulfate versus diazepam for eclampsia. Cochrane Database Syst Rev. 2010;12:CD000127.
18. Duley L, Henderson-Smart DJ, Chou D. Magnesium sulfate versus phenytoin for eclampsia. Cochrane Database Syst Rev. 2010;10:CD000128.
19. Duley L, Gulmezoglu AM, Chou D. Magnesium sulfate versus lytic cocktail for eclampsia. Cochrane Database Syst Rev. 2010;9:CD002960.
20. Mol BW, Roberts CT, Thangaratinam S, et al. Pre-eclampsia. Lancet. 2016;387(10022):999–1011. doi:10.1016/S0140-6736(15)00070-7.
21. Sibai BM. Preeclampsia and hypertension. In: Obstetrics: Normal and problem pregnancies. Ed. Steven G. Gabbe, Ed. Jennifer R. Niebyl, Ed. Joe Leigh Simpson, et al. Philadelphia: Elsevier, 2017;661–705.
22. Olsen-Chen C, Seligman NS. Hypertensive emergencies in pregnancy. Crit Care Clin. 2016;32:29–41.
23. Magee LA, Miremadi S, Li J, et al. Therapy with both magnesium sulfate and nifedipine does not increase the risk of serious magnesium-related maternal side effects in women with pre-eclampsia. Am J Obstet Gynecol. 2005;193:153–63.
24. Hohlagschwandtner M, Husslein P, Klebermass K, et al. Perinatal mortality and morbidity. Comparison between maternal transport, neonatal transport and inpatient antenatal treatment. Arch Gynecol Obstet. 2001;265:113.
25. Repke JT, Norwitz ER. Management of eclampsia. In: Hypertension in pregnancy. Ed. Alexander Heazell, Ed. Errol R. Norwitz, Ed. Louise C. Kenny, et al. New York: Cambridge Univsersity Press, 2011:141–158.
26. Matthews TJ, Menacker F, MacDorman MF. Infant mortality statistics from the 2000 period linked birth/infant death data set. Natl Vital Stat Rep. 2001;50:1.
27. Gabbe S, Niebyl J, et al. Obstetrics: normal and problem pregnancies. 2012. Chapter 35: hypertension.
28. Angelini D, Mahlmeister L. Liability in triage: management of EMTALA regulations and common obstetric risks. J Midwifery Womens Health. 2005;50(6):472–8.
29. Raps EC, et al. Delayed peripartum vasculopathy:cerebral eclampsia revisited. Ann Neurol. 1993;33:222–5.
30. Garg D, Rahaman B, Stein E, Dickman E. Late postpartum eclampsia with postpartum angiopathy: an uncommon diagnosis in the emergency department. J Emerg Med. 2015;49(6):e187–91.
31. Leitch C, Cameron A, Walker J. The changing pattern of eclampsia over a 60-year period. BJOG. 1997;104:917–22.
32. Chames M, Livingston J, Ivester T, et al. Late postpartum eclampsia: a preventable disease? Am J Obstet Gynecol. 2002;186:1174–7.
33. Matthys L, Coppage K, Lambers D, et al. Delayed postpartum preeclampsia: an experience of 151 cases. Am J Obstet Gynecol. 2004;190:1464–6.
34. Lubarsky S, Barton J, Friedman S, et al. Late postpartum eclampsia revisited. Obstet Gynecol. 1994;83:502–5.
35. Walters B, Thompson M, Lee A, et al. Blood pressure in the puerperium. Clin Sci. 1986;71:589–94.
36. Walters B, Walters T. Hypertension in the puerperium. Lancet. 1987;2:330.
37. Sibai BM. Etiology and management of postpartum hypertension-preeclampsia. Am J Obstet Gynecol. 2012:470–5.
38. Al-Safi Z, Imudia AN, Filetti LC, et al. Delayed postpartum preeclampsia and eclampsia: demographics, clinical course, and complications. Obstet Gynecol. 2011;118:1102–7.
39. Stella C, Jodicke C, How H, et al. Postpartum headache: Is your workup complete? Am J Obstet Gynecol. 2007;196:318–22.
40. Sibai B, Ramadan M, Usta I, et al. Maternal morbidity and mortality in 442 pregnancies with hemolysis, elevated liver enzymes and low platelets (HELLP syndrome). Am J Obstet Gynecol. 1993;169:1000–6.

41. Woudstra DM, Chandra S, Hofmeyr GJ, et al. Corticosteroids for HELLP (hemolysis, elevated liver enzymes, low platelets) syndrome in pregnancy. Cochrane Database Syst Rev. 2010(9). Art. No: CD008148.
42. Rahimpanah F, Smoleniec J. Partial mole, triploidy and proteinuric hypertension: two case reports. Aust N Z J Obstet Gynaecol. 2000;40:215–8.
44. Brittain PC, Bayliss P. Partial hydatidiform molar pregnancy presenting with severe pre-eclampsia prior to twenty weeks gestation: a case report and review of the literature. Mil Med. 1995;160:42–4.
45. Alsulyman OM, Castro MA, Zuckerman E, et al. Preeclampsia and liver infarction in early pregnancy associated with the antiphospholipid syndrome. Obstet Gynecol. 1996;88:644–6.
46. Craig K, Pinette MG, Blackstone J, et al. Highly abnormal maternal inhibin and beta-human chorionic gonadotropin levels along with severe HELLP (hemolysis, elevated liver enzymes, and low platelet count) syndrome at 17 weeks' gestation with triploidy. Am J Obstet Gynecol. 2000;182:737–9.
47. Nugent CE, Punch MR, Barr M, et al. Persistence of partial molar placenta and severe pre-eclampsia after selective termination in a twin pregnancy. Obstet Gynecol. 1996;87:829–31.
48. Hazra S, Waugh J, Bosio P. "Pure" preeclampsia before 20 weeks of gestation: a unique entity. BJOG. 2003;110:1034–5.
49. Imasawa T, Nishiwaki T, Nishimura M, et al. A case of "pure" preeclampsia with nephrotic syndrome before 15 weeks of gestation in a patient whose renal biopsy showed glomerular capillary endotheliosis. Am J Kidney Dis. 2006;48:495–501.
50. Sibai BM, Lindheimer M, Hauth J, et al. Risk factors for preeclampsia, abruptio placentae, and adverse neonatal outcomes among women with chronic hypertension. National Institute of Child Health and Human Development Network of Maternal-Fetal Medicine Units. N Engl J Med. 1998;339:667–71.
51. Ferrer RL, Sibai BM, Mulrow CD, et al. Management of mild chronic hypertension during pregnancy: a review. Obstet Gynecol. 2000;96:849–60.

Chapter 5
Bleeding in Late Pregnancy

Maria Dynin and David R. Lane

Introduction

Bleeding in late pregnancy is less common than in early pregnancy and often heralds serious and potentially life-threatening complications. Antepartum hemorrhage is defined as any vaginal bleeding in the second half of pregnancy but before birth, usually considered after 20 weeks' gestation. Antepartum bleeding complicates approximately 5% of pregnancies [1]. Major causes include "bloody show" associated with labor, placenta previa, placental abruption, and, rarely, uterine rupture and vasa previa. Massive acute hemorrhage and emergency operative delivery are associated with both maternal and fetal morbidity and mortality; therefore, evaluation must be swift and definitive. While late pregnancy complications are infrequently managed in the emergency department (ED), emergency physicians must be prepared to identify the source of late-trimester bleeding and to stabilize mother and fetus until definitive obstetric management can be obtained.

Emergency Department Evaluation

The initial assessment of vaginal bleeding in late pregnancy begins with obtaining maternal vital signs, determining gestational age and fetal well-being, and acquiring a clear history of the onset and description of bleeding. Bleeding that is sudden

M. Dynin, M.D. (✉)
Department of Emergency Medicine, MedStar Georgetown University Hospital, 3800
Reservoir Road NW, Washington, DC 20007, USA
e-mail: mydynin@gmail.com

D.R. Lane, M.D.
Department of Emergency Medicine, MedStar Southern Maryland Hospital Center,
7503 Surratts Road, Clinton, MD 20735, USA
e-mail: david.r.lane@medstar.net

© Springer International Publishing AG 2017
J. Borhart (ed.), *Emergency Department Management of Obstetric Complications*,
DOI 10.1007/978-3-319-54410-6_5

onset, painless, and bright red points toward placenta previa. Bleeding associated with pain, following trauma, or darker in color points toward placental abruption. Bleeding may vary from spotting to exsanguination.

The physical exam should include an abdominal and external uterus exam. Loss of normal uterine contour or the ability to palpate fetal parts indicates uterine rupture. A uterus that is tender, firm, or rigid may indicate placental abruption. An external genital and sterile speculum exam may be performed, but digital cervical exam is contraindicated until placenta previa has been excluded [2].

Laboratory tests may give helpful objective data to assess the extent of vaginal bleeding, though in acute hemorrhage, the data could be falsely reassuring. A complete blood count (CBC) should be ordered to evaluate for anemia, thrombocytopenia, and platelet consumption. A blood type and screen is required to determine Rh status and to prepare for potential blood transfusion. Women who are Rh negative should receive 300 mcg $Rh_o(D)$ immune globulin to prevent Rh alloimmunization. In cases of significant bleeding, prothrombin time (PT), partial thromboplastin time (PTT), and fibrinogen levels should be checked, as placenta abruption and uterine rupture may lead to disseminated intravascular coagulation (DIC). A basic metabolic panel, magnesium level, hepatic panel, and urinalysis with urine toxicology may also be considered if there is concern for preeclampsia or substance abuse.

Transabdominal or transvaginal obstetric ultrasound can be helpful to differentiate sources of late-trimester bleeding and should be performed to look for intrauterine and intra-abdominal bleeding, placenta location, and fetal movement.

Continuous fetal monitoring, if available, is highly recommended. Any decelerations and loss of variability on fetal heart rate tracings should be noted, yet some resolve with maternal resuscitation. Persistent decelerations may require emergent cesarean delivery even before the etiology of the hemorrhage is established.

In all cases of late pregnancy vaginal bleeding, an obstetrician should be consulted as early as possible. The ultimate management is based on maternal stability and gestational age. Most patients with late pregnancy bleeding will be admitted for observation and monitoring; those near term are often delivered.

Placenta Previa

Placenta previa is defined as placental implantation in the lower uterine segment, with either complete or partial obstruction of the cervical os [3]. The incidence of placenta previa varies from 3.5 to 4.6 per 1000 births [4]. Placenta previa is often found incidentally during routine second-trimester ultrasound. Previa is noted on about 4% of ultrasound studies performed at 20–24 weeks' gestation; however, at 37–42 weeks, it is present in only 0.4% of pregnancies [4, 5].

The exact pathogenesis of placenta previa is unknown and the condition appears to be multifactorial. There are a variety of reported risk factors placenta previa, including advanced maternal age (>35 years), infertility treatment, multiparity, multiple gestations, previous placenta previa, and pervious uterine surgery or cesarean delivery [4, 6–13].

The classic clinical presentation of placenta previa is sudden painless bright red vaginal bleeding. Emergency physicians should assume that a pregnant woman past 20 weeks gestation with painless vaginal bleeding has placenta previa until proven otherwise. The uterus usually remains soft, yet 10–20% of women may have associated uterine contractions [14, 15]. In about one-third of affected pregnancies, the initial bleeding episode occurs prior to 30 weeks' gestation [16].

Bleeding from placenta previa can range from minor to severe. In the absence of cervical instrumentation or cervical digital examination, the sentinel bleed usually is not sufficient to produce hemodynamic instability or to threaten fetal viability [17, 18]. The initial bleeding from placenta previa is thought to occur due to shearing forces between the inelastic placenta and the uterine wall, as gradual changes in the cervix and lower uterine segment lead to partial detachment. Bleeding is primarily thought to be from the maternal side of the placenta, as no fetal vessels are exposed in placenta previa. Sexual intercourse and vaginal exams can also cause bleeding from disruption of the intervillous space, which is the space between the fetal and maternal blood vessels. Because of this, digital cervical examination is contraindicated and should not be performed until placenta previa has been ruled out [1].

The diagnosis of placenta previa is made by ultrasound (Fig. 5.1). Transabdominal ultrasound (TAUS) is an appropriate initial study. However, several anatomical features can lead to inaccurate results such as a posteriorly located placenta, an overdistended bladder compressing the anterior lower uterine segment, and a low lying fetal head. Transvaginal ultrasonography (TVUS) has been shown to be more sensitive and specific for diagnosis of placenta previa [19–24]. One study demonstrated the superiority of TVUS as compared to the TAUS approach: false-positive and false-negative rates of TVUS were 1.0% and 2.0%, vs. 7% and 8%, for TAUS [19]. Similarly, another study found that landmarks were poorly seen in 50% of the cases using TAUS and a definitive diagnosis could not be made due to suboptimal visualization; subsequently, once TVUS was performed, the diagnosis changed in 26% of

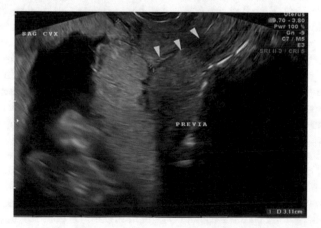

Fig. 5.1 Placenta previa. Ultrasound image showing placenta covering cervical os (*arrowheads*). Image courtesy of Ian Suchet

the cases [20]. TVUS can be safely performed in late pregnancy if the vaginal probe is placed 2–3 cm away from cervical os with optimal angle from os [21].

Management of placenta previa depends on gestational age and stability of the mother. Unstable patients require aggressive resuscitation with blood products and emergent cesarean section. For stable patients, the main goal is to prolong pregnancy until fetal lung maturity is adequate for delivery. Patients between 24 and 34 weeks gestation should be given corticosteroids to accelerate fetal lung maturity if delivery within 7 days is anticipated [25]. Forty-four percent of women with placenta previa deliver before 37 weeks [26]. An obstetrician should evaluate all patients with placenta previa. For the majority of patients, admission to an obstetric unit is required.

Placental Abruption

Placental abruption, also known as abruptio placentae, is defined as separation of the placenta from the uterine wall before delivery. This condition occurs in about 1% of all pregnancies, and about 50% of these occur prior to 36 weeks' gestation [27–29]. The presentation of placenta abruption can vary widely, making the diagnosis difficult. Placental abruption is the most common cause of intrapartum fetal death, with neonatal mortality ranging 10–30% of all abruption cases [29, 30]. Risk factors for abruptio placentae include maternal trauma, previous abruption, hypertension, cocaine use, multiparity, and advanced maternal age [29–34].

The classic presentation of placental abruption is the acute onset of abdominal pain with or without dark red vaginal bleeding. The hallmark of placental abruption is pain and tenderness, which is found in 70% of patients [33, 35]. The pain may be abdominal, pelvic, or back pain. Contractions in placental abruption are usually high frequency and low amplitude and result in pain worse between contractions [36]. The uterus tends to be firm and rigid, and hypertonia develops as the abruption expands.

Vaginal bleeding occurs in approximately 80–70% of patients with placental abruption [33, 35]. Bleeding can be light to hemorrhagic and may be bright red to dark burgundy. In abruption, maternal spiral arteries rupture, causing blood to accumulate and split the decidua from the uterine wall. A hematoma can develop without vaginal bleeding in 10–20% of abruptions [33]. These "concealed abruptions" are either early in the vessel bleeding phase or there is partial placental separation between the fetal membranes and decidua; hence, these patients present with preterm labor and abdominal pain. However, if bleeding continues, complete dissection of the uterine-placental interface can occur as the hematoma grows. Importantly, the amount of vaginal bleeding does not correlate with the severity of the abruption.

Placental abruption can quickly progress to hemorrhagic shock in the mother, and the lack of gas exchange and nutrients to the fetus causes fetal distress. Indeed, fetal distress is noted in 60% of patients with placenta abruption and may be the only sign that an abruption has occured [35]. When placental separation exceeds 50%, acute disseminated intravascular coagulation (DIC) is common and fetal death is almost certain [37].

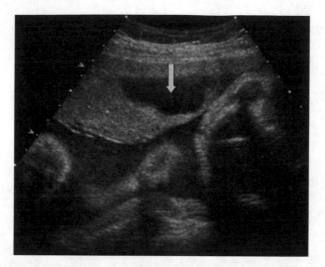

Fig. 5.2 Ultrasound image showing acute placental abruption with a retroplacental hematoma (*arrow*) lifting part of the placenta. Meguerdichian, D. "Complications in late pregnancy" Emergency Medicine Clinics of North America. Philadelphia, Elsevier. 2011. *Courtesy of* Carol Benson, MD, Brigham and Women's Hospital Department of Radiology, with permission

Placental abruption is a largely clinical diagnosis. Ultrasound may be used, as a hyperechoic clot or sign of bleeding posterior to the placenta, if visualized, is highly suggestive of placental abruption (Fig. 5.2). Unfortunately, these findings are only present in about 25% of cases [38]. While ultrasound cannot reliably exclude abruption, it can be used to exclude placenta previa.

Management of patients with abruptio placentae should begin with placement of two large bore IVs, resuscitation with intravenous fluids or blood products, reversal of any coagulopathies, and immediate obstetric consultation. Since DIC occurs in about 10% of placenta abruption cases, fibrinogen, PT, and PTT should be sent with standard labs [39]. Blood type and screen should also be sent if this diagnosis is suspected. In most cases of placental abruption, immediate delivery is necessary and tocolytics are contraindicated. One case-control study found that decision to deliver interval of 20 min or less resulted in better neonatal outcomes [40].

Vasa Previa

Vasa previa, from the Latin "vessels before the road," is the presence of fetal vessels between the cervix and the presenting fetal part. This is a very serious cause of vaginal bleeding in late pregnancy, with greater than 50% perinatal mortality [41]. Rupture of only 100 ml of exposed fetal vessels can cause fetal exsanguination or death [42]. Obstetric consultation should be obtained immediately. The condition is usually diagnosed in the second or third trimester by ultrasound (Fig. 5.3). The

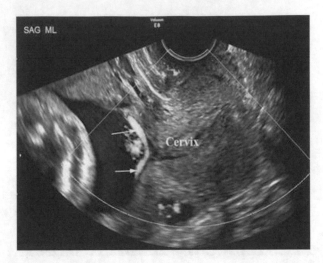

Fig. 5.3 Vasa previa. *Arrows* pointing to fetal vessels between the cervix and presenting fetal part. Image courtesy of Ian Suchet

incidence of vasa previa is about 1 in 2500 births, yet may be even higher in pregnancies resulting from assisted reproductive technologies [41]. The risk factors for vasa previa include placenta previa, in vitro fertilization, multiple gestations, and velamentous cord insertion (i.e., when the placental end of the umbilical cord consists of divergent umbilical vessels that are not protected by Wharton's jelly and are at risk for rupture) [41, 43, 44].

Patients with vasa previa tend to present with vaginal bleeding immediately after spontaneous rupture of membranes or amniotomy; it is rare for fetal vessels to rupture without rupture of membranes. Without a history of vasa previa on a prior ultrasound, this diagnosis should be suspected if there are fetal heart abnormalities accompanied with sudden vaginal bleeding after rupture of membranes. Fetal heart monitoring in this condition tends to present as sinusoidal or bradycardic pattern [43, 45]. Any non-reassuring fetal monitoring or unstable maternal vital signs is an indication for operative delivery. Upon delivery, focus should be placed on neonatal resuscitation due to the high mortality rate. If there is a reassuring fetal heart rate, stable maternal vital signs, and nonhemorrhagic vaginal bleeding, an Apt test (a qualitative test of vaginal bleeding to determine the absence or presence of fetal blood) may be performed to diagnose vasa previa [46].

Uterine Rupture

Uterine rupture is a life-threatening cause of vaginal bleeding in late pregnancy. The incidence depends on cause of rupture and is difficult to estimate. It is much more common in patients with history of previous cesarean sections, but is still possible in an unscarred uterus. In fact, 13% of uterine ruptures occur in unscarred uteruses, and this group has a higher morbidity and mortality compared to uterine rupture with a previously scarred uterus [47, 48]. One study found a perinatal mortality of 65% in the unscarred uterus [47]. In addition to history of previous cesarean section, risk factors for uterine rupture include trauma, high parity, advanced maternal age, and congenital disorders (e.g., Ehlers-Danlos) [47–54].

The classic presentation of uterine rupture is the sudden onset of abdominal pain, loss of uterine tone, change in uterine shape or contour, vaginal bleeding, and shock. A scarred uterus rupture may have a less severe onset presentation than that of an unscarred uterus due to previously altered vasculature [47]. Vaginal bleeding may be modest to hemorrhagic depending on the site of uterine rupture. These patients have a tender, boggy uterus on exam, and abdominal girth may quickly expand as blood accumulates. Fetal monitoring is more reliable than abdominal pain in diagnosing uterine rupture [53, 55–58]. Bradycardia is the most common finding on fetal monitoring, but no fetal heart rate pattern is pathognomonic [53, 55–58].

In any suspicion of uterine rupture, immediate resuscitation and surgical intervention are crucial. In the rare situations where there is only mild abdominal pain, stable fetal heart tracings, and light vaginal bleeding, an ultrasound exam may be performed. An abdomen or focused assessment with sonography for trauma (FAST) ultrasound exam with significant blood or defect in uterine wall can help reach the uterine rupture diagnosis. Studies have noted that a physician has about 10–37 min from frank uterine rupture to intervention before there is significant fetal and maternal morbidity [54, 56, 59]. Therefore, this is a diagnosis that should be immediately considered in antepartum hemorrhage.

Other Causes of Antepartum Hemorrhage

The previously discussed topics are some of the more concerning diagnoses of late-trimester vaginal bleeding, but there are numerous causes and degrees of vaginal bleeding in pregnancy. Vaginal and cervical sources of bleeding include vaginitis, cervicitis, warts, polyps, fissures, and trauma. Fibroids and circumvallate placenta are intrauterine causes of vaginal bleeding. Patients may have mild vaginal bleeding following cervical exams, sexual intercourse, or stripping of membranes by obstetricians near term. Most of these cases presents with spotting or minimal vaginal bleeding. Regardless, all patients with vaginal bleeding in late pregnancy should be evaluated with serious concern, and care should be managed in close consultation with an obstetrician.

Summary

Bleeding in late pregnancy can herald potentially life-threatening conditions such as placenta previa, placental abruption, vasa previa, or uterine rupture. These emergencies are infrequently managed in the ED and can be challenging for the entire team.

It is incumbent on the emergency physician to make a swift, accurate diagnosis and to lead resuscitative efforts. Obstetric consultation should be obtained as early as possible. Prompt, coordinated interdisciplinary care can be lifesaving for both the mother and fetus. Ultimately, management depends on maternal stability and gestational age; many patients will require emergent cesarean delivery.

Key Points

- A pregnant woman past 20 weeks gestation with sudden onset painless vaginal bleeding has placenta previa until proven otherwise.
- Digital cervical exams are contraindicated until placenta previa has been excluded.
- Placental abruption may present with or without vaginal bleeding; the amount of bleeding does not correlate with the severity of the abruption.
- Ultrasound is used to diagnose placenta previa; it cannot reliably exclude placental abruption.
- Obstetric consultation should be obtained early in the ED course of all patients with late pregnancy bleeding.

References

1. Hull AD, Resnick R. Placenta previa, placenta accreta, abruptio placentae, and vasa previa. In: Creasy RK, Resnick R, Iams JD, et al editors. Maternal-fetal medicine: Priniciple and practice. 7th ed. Philadelphia, PA: Elsevier Saunders, p. 732–42.
2. Chilaka VN, Konje JC, Clarke S, Taylor DJ. Practice observed: is speculum examination on admission a necessary procedure in the management of all cases of antepartum haemorrhage? J Obstet Gynaecol. 2000;20:396–8.
3. Silver RM. Abnormal placentation: placenta previa, vasa previa, and placenta accreta. Obstet Gynecol. 2015;126(3):654–68.
4. Faiz AS, Ananth CV. Etiology and risk factors for placenta previa: an overview and meta-analysis of observational studies. J Matern Fetal Neonatal Med. 2003;13:175–90.
5. Mustafa SA, Brizot ML, Carvalho MH, Watanabe L, Kahhale S, Zugaib M. Transvaginal ultrasonography in predicting placenta previa at delivery: a longitudinal study. Ultrasound Obstet Gynecol. 2002;20:356–9.
6. Marshall NE, Fu R, Guise JM. Impact of multiple cesarean deliveries on maternal morbidity: a systematic review. Am J Obstet Gynecol. 2011;205(3):262.
7. Ananth CV, Smulian JC, Vintzileos AM. The association of placenta previa with history of cesarean delivery and abortion: a metaanalysis. Am J Obstet Gynecol. 1997;177(5):1071.
8. Rasmussen S, Albrechtsen S, Dalaker K. Obstetric history and the risk of placenta previa. Acta Obstet Gynecol Scand. 2000;79(6):502–7.
9. Macones GA, Sehdev HM, Parry S, Morgan MA, Berlin JA. The association between maternal cocaine use and placenta previa. Am J Obstet Gynecol. 1997;177(5):1097–100.
10. Iyasu S, Saftlas AK, Rowley DL, Koonin LM, Lawson HW, Atrash HK. The epidemiology of placenta previa in the United States, 1979 through 1987. Am J Obstet Gynecol. 1993;168(5):1424–9.

11. Rosenberg T, Pariente G, Sergienko R, Wiznitzer A, Sheiner E. Critical analysis of risk factors and outcome of placenta previa. Arch Gynecol Obstet. 2011;284(1):47.
12. Ananth CV, Demissie K, Smulian JC, Vintzileos AM. Placenta previa in singleton and twin births in the United States, 1989 through 1998: a comparison of risk factor profiles and associated conditions. Am J Obstet Gynecol. 2003;188(1):275.
13. Sheiner E, Shoham-Vardi I, Hallak M, Hershkowitz R, Katz M, Mazor M. Placenta previa: obstetric risk factors and pregnancy outcome. Matern Fetal Med. 2001;10:414–9.
14. Cotton DB, Read JA, Paul RH, Quilligan EJ. The conservative aggressive management of placenta previa. Am J Obstet Gynecol. 1980;137(6):687.
15. Silver R, Depp R, Sabbagha RE, Dooley SL, Socol ML, Tamura RK. Placenta previa: aggressive expectant management. Am J Obstet Gynecol. 1984;150(1):15.
16. Dola CP, Garite TJ, Dowling DD, Friend D, Ahdoot D, Asrat T. Placenta previa: does its type affect pregnancy outcome? Am J Perinatol. 2003;20(7):353–60.
17. Sakornbut E, Leeman L, Fontaine P. Late pregnancy bleeding. Am Fam Physician. 2007;75(8):1199–206.
18. Abbrescia K, Sheridan B. Complications of second and third trimester pregnancies. Emerg Med Clin North Am. 2003;21(3):695–710.
19. Leerentveld RA, Gilberts EC, Arnold MJ, Wladimiroff JW. Accuracy and safety of transvaginal sonographic placental localization. Obstet Gynecol. 1990;(76):759–62.
20. Smith RS, Lauria MR, Comstock CH, Treadwell MC, Kirk JS, Lee W, Bottoms SF. Transvaginal ultrasonography for all placentas that appear to be low-lying or over the internal cervical os. Ultrasound Obstet Gynecol. 1997;9(1):22.
21. Timor-Tritsch IE, Yunis R. Confirming the safety of transvaginal sonography in patients suspected of placenta previa. Obstet Gynecol. 1993;81(5Pt 1):742.
22. Sunna E, Ziadeh S. Transvaginal and transabdominal ultrasound for the diagnosis of placenta praevia. J Obstet Gynaecol. 1999;19(2):152.
23. Sherman SJ, Carlson DE, Platt LD, Medearis AL. Transvaginal ultrasound: does it help in the diagnosis of placenta previa? Ultrasound Obstet Gynecol. 1992;2(4):256.
24. Oyelese KO, Holden D, Awadh A, Coates S, Campbell S. Placenta praevia: the case for transvaginal sonography. Contemp Rev Obstet Gynaecol. 1999;11:257–61.
25. Practice Bulletin No. 159: Management of preterm labor. Obstet Gynecol. 2016;127:29–38.
26. Bose DA, Assel BG, Hill JB, Chauhan SP. Maintenance tocolytics for preterm symptomatic placenta previa: a review. Am J Perinatol. 2011;28(1):45–50.
27. Hladky K, Yankowitz J, Hansen WF. Placental abruption. Obstet Gynecol Surv. 2002;57:299–305.
28. Rasmussen S, Irgens LM, Bergsjo P, Dalaker K. The occurrence of placental abruption in Norway 1967–1991. Acta Obstet Gynecol Scand. 1996;75:222–8.
29. Tikkanen M. Placental abruption: epidemiology, risk factors and consequences. Acta Obstet Gynecol Scand. 2011;90(2):140–9.
30. Kyrklund-Blomberg NB, Gennser G, Cnattingius S. Placental abruption and perinatal death. Paediatr Perinat Epidemiol. 2001;15(3):290–7.
31. Abu-Heija A. Abruptio placentae: risk factors and perinatal outcome. J Obstet Gynaecol Res. 1998;24(2):141–4.
32. Ananth CV, Smulian JC, Demissie K, Vintzileos AM, Knuppel RA. Placental abruption among singleton and twin births in the United States: risk factor profiles. Am J Epidemiol. 2001;153(8):771.
33. Oyelese Y, Ananth CV. Placental abruption. Obstet Gynecol. 2006;108(4):1005–16.
34. Mbah AK, Alio AP, Fombo DW, Bruder K, Dagne G, Salihu HM. Association between cocaine abuse in pregnancy and placenta-associated syndromes using propensity score matching approach. Early Hum Dev. 2012;88(6):333–7.
35. Tikkanen M, Nuutila M, Hiilesmaa V, et al. Clinical presentation and risk factors of placental abruption. Acta Obstet Gynecol Scand. 2006;85(6):700–5.
36. Yeo L, Ananth C, et al. Glob. libr. women's med., (ISSN: 1756–2228). 2008.
37. Ananth CV, Berkowitz GS, Savitz DA, et al. Placental abruption and adverse perinatal outcomes. JAMA. 1999;282:1646–51.

38. Glantz C, Purnell L. Clinical utility of sonography in the diagnosis and treatment of placental abruption. J Ultrasound Med. 2002;21:837–40.
39. Witlin AG, Sibai BM. Perinatal and maternal outcome following abruptio placentae. Hypertens Pregnancy. 2001;20:195–203.
40. Kayani SI, Walkinshaw SA, Preston C. Pregnancy outcome in severe placental abruption. BJOG. 2003;110:679–83.
41. Oyalese KO, Turner M, Lees C, Campbell S. Vasa previa: an avoidable obstetric tragedy. Obstet Gynecol Surv. 1999;54:138–45.
42. Lubin B. Neonatal anaemia secondary to blood loss. Clin Haematol. 1978;7:19–34.
43. Society of Maternal-Fetal (SMFM) Publications Committee, Sinkey RG, Odibo AO, Dashe JS. #37: Diagnosis and management of vasa previa. Am J Obstet Gynecol. 2015;213(5):615.
44. Hasegawa J, Nakamura M, Sekizawa A, Matsuoka R, Ichizuka K, Okai T. Prediction of risk for vasa previa at 9-13 weeks' gestation. J Obstet Gynaecol Res. 2011;37(10):1346–51.
45. Kruitwagen RF, Nijhuis JG. Ruptured vasa praevia complicated by a sinusoidal fetal heart rate pattern: a case report. Eur J Obstet Gynecol Reprod Biol. 1991;39:147–50.
46. Odunsi K, Bullough CH, Henzel J, Polanska A. Evaluation of chemical tests for fetal bleeding from vasa previa. Int J Gynaecol Obstet. 1996;55(3):207.
47. Gibbins KJ, Weber T, Holmgren CM, Porter TF, Varner MW, Manuck TA. Maternal and fetal morbidity associated with uterine rupture of the unscarred uterus. Am J Obstet Gynecol. 2015;213(3):382.
48. Zwart JJ, Richters JM, Ory F, de Vries JI, Bloemenkamp KW, van Roosmalen J. Uterine rupture in The Netherlands: a nationwide population-based cohort study. BJOG. 2009;116(8):1069.
49. Al-Zirqi I, Daltveit AK, Forsen L, et al. Risk factors for complete uterine rupture. Am J Obstet Gynecol. 2017;216(2):165e1–165e8
50. Rageth JC, Juzi C, Grossenbacher H. Delivery after previous cesarean: a risk evaluation. Swiss Working Group of Obstetric and Gynecologic Institutions. Obstet Gynecol. 1999;93(3):332–7.
51. Rudd NL, Nimrod C, Holbrook KA, Byers PH. Pregnancy complications in type IV Ehlers-Danlos Syndrome. Lancet. 1983;1(8314–5):50.
52. National Institutes of Health Consensus Development Conference Panel. National Institutes of Health Consensus Development conference statement: vaginal birth after cesarean: new insights March 8–10, 2010. Obstet Gynecol. 2010;115(6):127.
53. Ozdemir I, Yucel N, Yucel O. Rupture of the pregnant uterus: a 9-year review. Arch Gynecol Obstet. 2005;272(3):229.
54. Bujold E, Gauthier RJ. Neonatal morbidity associated with uterine rupture: what are the risk factors? Am J Obstet Gynecol. 2002;186(2):311–4.
55. Bujold E, Mehta SH, Bujold C, Gauthier RJ. Interdelivery interval and uterine rupture. Am J Obstet Gynecol. 2002;187(5):1199–202.
56. Leung AS, Leung EK, Paul RH. Uterine rupture after previous cesarean delivery: maternal and fetal consequences. Am J Obstet Gynecol. 1993;169(4):945–50.
57. Rodriguez MH, Masaki DI, Phelan JP, Diaz FG. Uterine rupture: are intrauterine pressure catheters useful in the diagnosis? Am J Obstet Gynecol. 1989;161(3):666–9.
58. Johnson C, Oriol N. The role of epidural anesthesia in trial of labor. Reg Anesth. 1990;15(6):304–8.
59. Blanchette H, Blanchette M, McCabe J, Vincent S. Is vaginal birth after cesarean safe? Experience at a community hospital. Am J Obstet Gynecol. 2001;184(7):1478–87.

Chapter 6
Premature Rupture of Membranes and Preterm Labor

Eric Wei, Lili Sheibani, and Brian Sharp

Introduction

Premature rupture of membranes (PROM) and preterm labor are challenging obstetric complications for any emergency physician. In the United States, preterm delivery complicates approximately one in ten births and is the cause of at least 75% of neonatal deaths, not including congenital malformations. When preterm premature rupture of membranes occurs, several complications can occur including infection, premature delivery, placental abruption, and umbilical cord prolapse.

Complications of late pregnancy including PROM and preterm labor are infrequently managed in the emergency department (ED). Many hospitals have protocols where these patients are triaged directly to a labor and delivery (L&D) unit for further management by an obstetrician. However, an obstetrician or L&D unit may not always be immediately available and emergency physicians must be comfortable initially managing these complications. The rate of fetal and maternal morbidity can be reduced with accurate diagnosis of PROM and preterm labor, intervention to delay preterm delivery, timely administration of corticosteroids, and in certain cases, magnesium sulfate and antibiotics.

E. Wei, M.D., M.B.A. (✉)
Department of Emergency Medicine, LAC+USC Medical Center,
2051 Marengo Street, C2K115, Los Angeles, CA 90033, USA
e-mail: EWei@dhs.lacounty.gov

L. Sheibani, M.D.
Division of Maternal-Fetal Medicine, Department of Obstetrics and Gynecology, Keck School of Medicine, USC, 2020 Zonal Avenue, IRD 234, Los Angeles, CA 90033, USA

B. Sharp, M.D., F.A.C.E.P.
BerbeeWalsh Department of Emergency Medicine, University of Wisconsin,
800 University Bay Drive, Madison, WI 53705, USA
e-mail: bsharp@medicine.wisc.edu

© Springer International Publishing AG 2017   63
J. Borhart (ed.), *Emergency Department Management of Obstetric Complications*,
DOI 10.1007/978-3-319-54410-6_6

Preterm Premature Rupture of Membranes

Premature rupture of membranes (PROM) is rupture of membranes before labor. Preterm PROM refers to the rupture of membrane before labor that occurs prior to 37 weeks of gestation. Preterm PROM complicates approximately 3% of all pregnancies in the United States [1]. During pregnancy, the amniotic membrane protects the fetus from infection while providing an environment that allows for both growth and movement. Fluid exchange is facilitated in part by fetal swallowing and urination. The fetal airway contains a secreted fluid that allows for fetal breathing and promotes respiratory development.

Membrane rupture may occur for several reasons. At term it occurs due to normal physiologic weakening of membranes, while preterm membrane rupture can occur for several pathologic conditions [2, 3]. At earlier gestational age, one of the most common reasons is intraamniotic infection [4]. A previous history of preterm PROM is a risk factor for either preterm PROM or preterm labor in future pregnancies. Other risk factors include short cervical length, history of vaginal bleeding during pregnancy, low socioeconomic status, cigarette smoking, and illicit drug use [5, 6]. Other cases may be without any identifiable risk factors.

Labor is the ideal result of ruptured membranes at term; however, when the fetus is preterm, labor that often follows membrane rupture is problematic given the associated fetal complications of prematurity.

Emergency Department Evaluation

Initial evaluation of the patient presenting with preterm PROM includes determination of duration, amount, and persistence of fluid leakage. Classically, patients report a sudden gush of fluid with continuous leakage. If the clinical history is unclear, patients should be asked questions about recent vaginal or cervical infections, recent sexual activity, douching, and previous pelvic surgery.

The next step in diagnosis is determining the gestational age of the pregnancy based on patient's reported last menstrual period (LMP) or previous ultrasonography scans. If the patient is unable to report either menstrual or ultrasound dating, an ultrasound can be obtained in the emergency department to determine gestational age. Ultrasounds become less accurate for obstetric dating with advancing gestational age. As a general rule, ultrasound dating has an accuracy of +/− 2 weeks in the second trimester and +/− 3 weeks in the third trimester [7]. In addition to estimating gestational age, obstetric ultrasound is indicated in order to determine the fetal presentation, an estimated fetal weight, and amount of amniotic fluid. Oligohydramnios, defined as amniotic fluid index (AFI) ≤5 cm, may be present in PROM, but is not diagnostic.

Examination of patients with possible PROM should be performed under sterile conditions with a sterile speculum to minimize the risk of introduction of infection.

Table 6.1 Testing for PROM

Method	Result
Nitrazine	Amniotic fluid pH 7.1–7.3 turns nitrazine paper yellow; >7.3 is blue
Ferning	Amniotic fluid crystallizes and appears like a fern, identified under microscope
Pooling on speculum exam	Amniotic fluid collects in the posterior vaginal vault
Ultrasonography (not diagnostic)	Oligohydramnios (defined as AFI <5)

Avoid direct digital examination of the cervix in women with PROM because the risk of infection has been shown to be proportional to the number of digital examinations [8]. Table 6.1 lists the components of diagnosing PROM. At speculum examination, the diagnosis is confirmed by visualization of passing of fluid from the endocervical canal into the vagina and/or a "pool" of fluid in the posterior vaginal vault. Having the patient cough or applying gentle fundal pressure may assist in visualizing the passage of fluid. If in doubt, the fluid can be tested via nitrazine test for pH. The pH of normal vaginal fluid is 4.5–6, while amniotic fluid pH is 7.1–7.3 Blood or semen contamination, alkaline antiseptics, and bacterial vaginosis can increase the vaginal pH and lead to a false-positive nitrazine test. Vaginal fluid may also be applied to a microscope slide and examined for the presence of ferning. During the speculum exam, the physician should visualize the cervix and assess for dilation and effacement and look for any presenting fetal parts or umbilical cord prolapse. Cultures for group B streptococcus, chlamydia, and gonorrhea can also be collected during the speculum examination.

Management

Once the diagnosis of PROM is established, the management depends on the gestational age and maturity of the fetus. Important factors include whether or not labor is present and if there is suspected intraamniotic infection. All patients with preterm PROM should be evaluated for intraamniotic infection (chorioamnionitis). Chorioamnionitis occurs when vaginal or cervical bacteria ascend into the amniotic cavity and initiate an inflammation of the chorion and amnion. Risk factors include prolonged labor, PROM, and excessive digital examinations. Chorioamnionitis occurs in 15–25% of women with preterm PROM [9]. The incidence of infection is higher with earlier gestational age [4]. Table 6.2 lists diagnostic criteria for chorioamnionitis

The management of preterm PROM includes administration of antibiotics to reduce neonatal and maternal infections and to prolong the latency period (time from membrane rupture to delivery). There are several antibiotic regimens that have shown benefit. The regimen described by the American College of Obstetricians and Gynecologists (ACOG) in a 2016 practice bulletin is a 7-day antibiotic course

Table 6.2 Diagnosis of chorioamnionitis (typically fever plus two other signs)

Maternal signs and symptoms
Fever (>100.4 °F)
Tachycardia (>100/min)
Malodorous vaginal discharge
Fundal tenderness
Leukocytosis
Fetal signs
Fetal tachycardia (>160/min)
Decreases in variability on fetal heart rate monitoring

starting with intravenous ampicillin (2 g every 6 h) and oral erythromycin (250 mg every 6 h) for 48 h, followed by oral amoxicillin (250 mg every 8 h) and erythromycin base (333 mg every 8 h) [10]. Intrapartum antibiotic prophylaxis against group B streptococcus is also indicated for women with preterm PROM at risk for preterm delivery whose carrier status is unknown.

With regards to fetal lung maturity, a fetus beyond 36 weeks is very likely to have reached lung maturity. In a fetus before 36 weeks, administration of corticosteroids can accelerate lung maturity. Corticosteroids have the additional benefits of reducing neonatal mortality, respiratory distress syndrome, intraventricular hemorrhage, and necrotizing enterocolitis [11–13]. Previous studies have suggested increased risk of infection with administration of corticosteroids in the setting of preterm PROM, but larger studies have not supported these findings. A common regimen is intramuscular betamethasone 12 mg every 24 h for 2 days [14]. Completion of one course of corticosteroids is indicated, irrespective of membrane status, for pregnant women between 24 0/7 weeks and 34 0/7 weeks if there is a concern for premature delivery within 7 days [15].

Complications

Complications associated with preterm PROM include active preterm labor with malpresentation of fetus (breech presentation being the most common), umbilical cord prolapse, infection, fetal distress, and placental abruption (2–5% of pregnancies) [16]. After preterm PROM, infection and umbilical cord accidents contribute to 1–2% of fetal demise [17]. The most significant risks to the fetus after preterm PROM are the myriad of complications of prematurity, the most common being respiratory distress. Additionally, preterm PROM with intrauterine inflammation has been associated with increased risk of impaired neurodevelopment [18]. In approximately 50% of preterm PROM, birth will occur within 1 week [10]. Latency after membrane rupture is inversely correlated to gestational age at rupture of membranes. Obstetric consultation should be obtained early in the ED course of a patient with PROM or preterm PROM. Once fetal viability has been reached (>23 weeks), hospitalization is recommended for patients with PROM and preterm PROM.

Preterm Labor

Preterm birth is the leading cause of neonatal mortality and one of the most common reasons for hospitalization [19]. In the United States, approximately 12% of all births occur before term, and preterm labor preceded about 50% of these births [20, 21]. Preterm birth accounts for 70% of neonatal deaths and 36% of infant deaths as well as 25–50% of long-term neurologic impairment in children [22].

Preterm birth is defined as birth between 20 0/7 weeks of gestation and 36 6/7 weeks of gestation. In order to more accurately describe deliveries that occur at or beyond 37 0/7 weeks, new obstetric guidelines have more clearly designated early term as 37 to 38 6/7 weeks and full term as 39 0/7 weeks of gestation through 40 6/7 weeks of gestation [23]. The risk of poor birth outcomes generally decreases with advancing gestational age. The risk is highest for infants born before 34 weeks; however, even infants born between 34 and 37 weeks are more likely to have delivery complications, long-term impairment, and early death than those born later in pregnancy [19]. The risks of perinatal, neonatal, and infant morbidity and mortality are lowest for infants born between 39 0/7 weeks of gestation and 40 6/7 weeks of gestation [24, 25]. Spontaneous preterm birth includes birth that follows preterm labor, preterm PROM, and cervical insufficiency, but does not include indicated preterm delivery for either maternal or fetal condition.

Risk Factors

Identifying women who will give birth preterm is an inexact process and can be very challenging as the causes of preterm birth are not well understood. One of the biggest risk factors for preterm birth is a prior preterm birth, which increases a woman's risk by about twofold [23]. Another risk factor is short cervical length as measured by transvaginal ultrasound [26]. In most studies this is defined by cervix less than 2.5 cm up to 24 weeks gestational age, and in some studies up to 28 weeks [27]. Other risk factors for preterm birth include demographic factors, current pregnancy complications, substance abuse, uterine anomalies, iatrogenic complications, infections, and psychosocial stressors (Table 6.3). Additionally, some studies have linked previous uterine or cervical instrumentation to preterm labor.

Diagnosis

The diagnosis of preterm labor is usually based on clinical criteria of regular contractions accompanied by cervical dilation, effacement, or both before 37 weeks of gestation. It can also be defined by initial presentation of regular contractions and cervical dilation of at least 2 cm. Less than 10% of women who present with these

Table 6.3 Risk factors for preterm birth

Demographic:
Extremes of age (>40 or teenager)
Low socioeconomic status
Substance abuse (tobacco, cocaine)
Psychosocial stressors
Reproductive:
Prior preterm delivery
Uterine anomalies
Cervical incompetence
Placental abruption
Vaginal bleeding in pregnancy
Infectious:
Urinary tract infections
Non-uterine infections
Vaginal infections (bacterial vaginosis)

clinical findings actually give birth within 7 days of presentation [28]. Some of the early maternal signs of preterm labor include increase or change in vaginal discharge, pain from uterine contractions (sometimes reported as lower back pain), pelvic pressure, vaginal bleeding, and leakage of fluid.

Once cervical change and uterine contractions are present, the determination of prematurity is based on patient's reported LMP or gestational age determined by prior ultrasound. If there was no prenatal care, an ED ultrasound may assist in obtaining an estimated gestational age. In general, a fetus measuring less than 2500 grams on ultrasound is likely to be premature. To differentiate false labor (Braxton Hicks contractions) from true labor, uterine contraction monitoring and repeat cervical exam are used.

Management of Preterm Labor

The initial ED evaluation of a woman with possible premature labor includes urinalysis, complete blood count, type and screen, and ultrasonography. If delivery is not imminent, and an L&D unit is immediately available, these can be completed once the patient is transported. Intravenous hydration with 1–2 L of Lactated Ringers may assist with resolution of irregular contractions, although it is not an effective treatment for true preterm labor. Bed rest is indicated until diagnosis is clear. Additionally, any underlying causes for preterm contractions such as urinary tract infections should be treated.

The management of preterm labor hinges on the gestational age of the fetus and stability of the mother. If the fetus is viable and the mother is stable, the goal is to prolong pregnancy for up to 48 h to allow for corticosteroid treatment and safe transfer of the patient. This is accomplished with the use of tocolytics [29].

Tocolytics may be initiated in the ED in close consultation with an obstetrician to attempt to halt preterm labor

Several tocolytic agents have been used to inhibit contractions, and beta-adrenergic receptor agonists, calcium channel blockers, and nonsteroidal anti-inflammatory drugs (NSAIDs) are all considered first-line medications [30, 31]. Two of the most commonly used are nifedipine (calcium channel blocker) and indomethacin (NSAID). Because of potential maternal complications, beta-adrenergic receptor agonists and calcium channel blockers should be used with caution in combination with magnesium sulfate. Antenatal indomethacin has been associated with fetal necrotizing enterocolitis in some studies.

Only women with fetuses that would benefit from a 48-h delay in delivery should receive tocolytic treatment. Women with contractions but without cervical change should not be treated with tocolytics, and tocolytics are generally not indicated before fetal viability. Other contraindications include maternal or fetal distress, eclampsia, and preterm PROM (Table 6.4). The upper limit of tocolytic use is 34 weeks.

Magnesium sulfate was previously administered as a tocolytic, but now it is used mostly for fetal neuroprotection if birth is anticipated before 32 weeks. Clinical trials of magnesium sulfate for neuroprotection suggest that the predelivery administration reduces the occurrence of cerebral palsy [32]. None of the trials demonstrated significant prolongation of pregnancy when magnesium sulfate was given for neuroprotection. Hospitals that elect to use magnesium sulfate usually have protocols for its usage including administration regimen, concurrent tocolysis, and monitoring.

The single most beneficial intervention for improvement of neonatal outcomes among preterm births is antenatal corticosteroids. A single course is recommended for women between 24 0/7 weeks and 34 0/7 weeks of gestation and may be considered for pregnant women starting at 23 weeks who are at risk of delivery within 7 days. Corticosteroids are considered routine for all preterm deliveries because of the associated decreased neonatal morbidity and mortality [11, 33]. Neonates that receive corticosteroids have lower rates of respiratory distress syndrome, intracranial hemorrhage, necrotizing enterocolitis, and death.

A single repeat course of antenatal corticosteroids should be considered in women whose prior course was at least 7 days previously and who remain at risk for delivery at less than 34 weeks. A recent randomized controlled trial has suggested benefit in corticosteroids from 34–37 weeks in setting of late preterm birth [34]. The decision to give corticosteroids should be made in consultation with an obstetrician.

Table 6.4 Contraindications to tocolysis	
	Intrauterine fetal demise
	Lethal fetal anomaly
	Nonreassuring fetal status
	Severe preeclampsia or eclampsia
	Maternal bleeding with hemodynamic instability
	Chorioamnionitis
	Maternal contraindication
	ACOG Practice Bulletin 159

The most commonly used corticosteroids are betamethasone and dexamethasone. The treatment for a primary or rescue course should consist of either two 12-mg dose of betamethasone given intramuscularly 24 h apart or four 6-mg doses of dexamethasone every 12 h administered intramuscularly [35]. The first dose should be given even if delivery is likely before the second dose can be administered, as there is evidence showing benefit of even a single dose.

Antibiotics and Preterm Labor

Several maternal infections have been associated with preterm labor. Most studies have failed to demonstrate that antibiotics have any benefit of preventing preterm birth, respiratory distress syndrome, or neonatal sepsis. Nevertheless, maternal infections identified in the ED should be treated. This is distinct from using antibiotics for preterm PROM and group B streptococci carriers [36, 37]. If the group B streptococci status of a woman is unknown and delivery is anticipated, antibiotics to prevent group B streptococcus in the neonate should be initiated. Penicillin remains the drug of choice and ampicillin is an acceptable alternative. Erythromycin is no longer recommended due to resistance. If there is severe allergic reaction to penicillin (anaphylaxis), cefazolin may be administered. All antibiotics for group B streptococcus prophylaxis should be given intravenously [37].

Disposition

In many cases, patients presenting to the ED in preterm labor can be safely transported to a L&D unit for further management by an obstetrician. Because of the high risk associated with delivery outside an obstetric unit, the emergency physician should make every effort to arrange transport to a facility with both obstetric and neonatal resources if time allows. In the setting of preterm birth, the infant may require intensive care services immediately after delivery. Obstetric consultation should be sought early in the ED course of any patient in preterm labor. Some births are precipitous, and an obstetrician or L&D unit may not be immediately available. Emergency physicians must be prepared to deliver a premature infant and resuscitate mother and baby as necessary.

Summary

Preterm delivery occurs in approximately 12% of all births in the United States and contributes to significant perinatal morbidity and mortality. Preterm PROM can complicate a portion of the preterm deliveries. Diagnosis of preterm labor and preterm PROM can be initiated in the emergency department in consultation with an obstetrician. In all patients with preterm PROM, gestational age, fetal presentation, and fetal well-being should be determined. The emergency physician should evaluate for intrauterine infection, placental abruption, and fetal compromise.

Almost all cases of preterm PROM, PROM, and preterm labor will warrant admission to an obstetrics unit. The ultimate obstetric management depends on gestational age and risks of delivery versus risks of expectant management. Corticosteroids are recommended for pregnant women with anticipated preterm delivery and tocolytic treatment can be used for short-term prolongation of pregnancy (up to 48 h). In cases of imminent delivery, determination of fetal position is of utmost importance. Intravenous magnesium sulfate is recommended to reduce the severity and risk of cerebral palsy in infants if administered when birth is anticipated before 32 weeks. If delivery is anticipated and the group B streptococcus status is unknown, antibiotics should be initiated for prophylaxis.

Key Points

- Speculum exam to rule out PROM should be done under sterile technique.
- Direct digital examination should be avoided in PROM unless delivery seems imminent.
- The single most beneficial intervention for improvement of neonatal outcomes among preterm births is antenatal corticosteroids.
- A single course of corticosteroids are recommended for women between 24 0/7 and 34 0/7 weeks gestational age who are at risk for preterm delivery within 7 days.
- Magnesium sulfate is used for fetal neuroprotection if birth is anticipated before 32 0/7 weeks and reduces the risk of cerebral palsy in infants. Tocolytics can be used for up to 48 h to allow for corticosteroids
- A 7-day course of antibiotic therapy is indicated in women with preterm PROM less than 34 0/7 weeks.

References

1. Waters TP, Mercer B. Preterm PROM: prediction, prevention, principles. Clin Obstet Gynecol. 2011;54:307–12.
2. Moore RM, Mansour JM, Redline RW, et al. The physiology of fetal membrane rupture: insight gained from the determination of physical properties. Placenta. 2006;27:1037–51.
3. Mercer BM. Preterm premature rupture of the membranes. Obstet Gynecol. 2003;101:178–93.
4. Garite TJ, Freean RK. Chorioamnionitis in the preterm gestation. Obstet Gynecol. 1982;59:539–45.
5. Mercer BM, Goldenberg RL, Meis PJ, et al. The Preterm Prediction Study: prediction of preterm premature rupture of membranes through clinical findings and ancillary testing. The National Institute of Child Health and Human Development Maternal-Fetal Medicine Units Network. Am J Obstet Gynecol. 2000;183:738–45.

6. Harger JH, Hsing AW, Tuomala RE, et al. Risk factors for preterm premature rupture of membranes: a multicenter case-control study. Am J Obstet Gynecol. 1990;163:130–7.
7. Method for estimating due date. Committee opinion No. 611. American College of Obstetricians and Gynecologists. Obstet Gynecol. 2014;124: 863–6.
8. Alexander JM, Mercer BM, Miodovnik M, et al. The impact of digital cervical examinations on expectantly managed preterm rupture of membranes. Am J Obstet Gynecol. 2000;1003:183.
9. Kenyon S, Boulvain M, Neilson JP. Antibiotics for preterm rupture of membranes. Cochrane Database Syst Rev. 2010;(8). Art. No.: CD001058. DOI: 10.1002/14651858.CD001058.pub2.
10. Practice Bulletin No. 160: premature rupture of membranes. Obstet Gynecol. 2016;127:39–51.
11. Roberts D, Dalziel SR. Antenatal corticosteroids for accelerating fetal lung maturation for women at risk of preterm birth. Cochrane Database Syst Rev. 2006;(3). Art. No.:CD004454. Doi: 10.1002/14651858.
12. Vidaeff AC, Ramin SM. Antenatal corticosteroids after preterm premature rupture of membranes. Clin Obstet Gynecol. 2011;54:337–43.
13. Harding JE, Pang J, Knight DB, Liggins GC. Do antenatal corticosteroids help in the setting of preterm rupture of membranes? Am J Obstet Gynecol. 2001;184:131–9.
14. Effect of corticosteroids for fetal maturation on perinatal outcomes. NIH Consens Statement. 1994;12:1–24.
15. Practice Bulletin No. 159: management of preterm labor. Obstet Gynecol. 2016;127:29–38
16. Ananth CV, Oyelese Y, Srinivas N, et al. Preterm premature rupture of membranes, intrauterine infection, and oligohydramnios: risk factors for placenta abruption. Obstet Gynecol. 2004;104:71–7.
17. Mercer BM, Arheart KL. Antimicrobial therapy in expectant management of preterm premature rupture of the membranes. Lancet. 1996;347:410.
18. Yoon BH, Romero R, Park JS, Kim CJ, Kim SH, Choi JH, et al. Fetal exposure to an intra-amniotic inflammation and the development of cerebral palsy at the age of three years. Am J Obstet Gynecol. 2000;182:675–81.
19. Martin JA, Hamilton BE, Sutton PD, Ventura SJ, Mathews TJ, Osterman MJ. Births: final data for 2008. Natl Vital Stat Rep. 2010;59:1–72.
20. Simhan NH, Iams JD, Romero R. Preterm birth. In: Gabbe SG, Niebyl JR, Simpson JL, Landon MB, Galan HL, Jauniaux ER, et al., editors. Obstetrics: normal and problems pregnancies. 6th ed. Philadelphia, PA: Elsevier Saunders; 2012. p. 628–56.
21. Martin JA, Hamilton BE, Ventura SJ, et al. Births: final data for 2009. Natl Vital Stat Rep. 2011;60:1–71.
22. Spong CY. Prediction and prevention of recurrent spontaneous preterm birth. Obstet Gynecol. 2007;110:405–15.
23. Definition of term pregnancy. Committee Opinion No. 579. American College of Obstetricians and Gynecologists. Obstet Gynecol. 2013;122:1139–40.
24. Clark SL, Miller DD, Belfort MA, et al. Neonatal and maternal outcomes associated with elective term delivery. Am J Obstet Gynecol. 2009;200:156.e1–4.
25. Fleishman AR, Oinuma M, Clark SL. Rethinking the definition of "term pregnancy.". Obstet Gynecol. 2010;116:136–9.
26. Mella MT, Berghella V. Prediction of preterm birth: cervical sonography. Semin Perinatol. 2009;33:317–24.
27. Crane JM, Hutchens D. Transvaginal sonographic measurement of cervical length to predict preterm birth in asymptomatic women at increased risk: a systematic review. Ultrasound Obstet Gynecol. 2008;31:579–87.
28. Bakketeig LS, Hoffman HJ. Epidemiology of preterm birth: results from a longitudinal study of births in Norway. In: Elder MG, Hendricks CH, editors. Preterm labor. Boston, MA: Butterworths; 1981. p. 17–46.
29. Practice Bulletin No. 130: prediction and prevention of preterm birth. Obstet Gynecol. 2012;120:964–73.

30. King JF, Flenady V, Paptsonis D, et al. Calcium channel blockers for inhibiting preterm labour. Cochrane Database Syst Rev. 2003;(1). Art. No.:CD002255. Doi: 10.1002/14651858.
31. King JF, Flenady V, Cole S, Thornton S. Cyclooxygenase (COX) inhibitors for treating preterm labour. Cochrane Database Syst Rev. 2005;(2). Art. No.:CD001992. Doi: 10.1002/14651858. CD001992.pub2.
32. Conde-Agudelo A, Romero R. Antenatal magnesium sulfate for the prevention of cerebral palsy in preterm infants less than 34 weeks' gestation: a systematic review and meta-analysis. Am J Obstet Gynecol. 2009;200:595–609.
33. Antenatal corticosteroids revisited: repeat courses: NIH Consens Statement. 2000;17(2):1–18.
34. Gyamfi-Bannerman C, Thorn EA, Blackwell SC, et al. Antenatal betamethasone for women at risk for late preterm delivery. N Engl J Med. 2016;375:486–7.
35. Antenatal corticosteroids therapy for fetal maturation. Committee Opinion No. 475. American College of Obstetricians and Gynecologists. Obstet Gynecol 2011;117:422–4.
36. Prevention of perinatal group B streptococcal disease—revisited guidelines from CDC, 2010. Division of Bacterial Diseases, National Center for Immunization and Respiratory Diseases. MMWR. Recomm Rep. 2010;59(RR-10):1–36.
37. Prevention of early-onset group B streptococcal disease in newborns. Committee Opinion No. 485. American College of Obstetricians and Gynecologists. Obstet Gynecol. 2011;117:1019–27.

Chapter 7
Precipitous Labor and Emergency Department Delivery

Brian Sharp, Kristen Sharp, and Eric Wei

Introduction

Every year in the United States, hundreds of patients deliver precipitously in the emergency department (ED). While the vast majority has good outcomes, ED deliveries can be extremely stressful and chaotic. These rare events must be approached with a calm mind and a methodological approach. It is also important that emergency physicians are prepared for management of the various complications that can arise including shoulder dystocia, prolapsed umbilical cord, and breech delivery.

Labor is divided into three stages. Stage 1 involves a latent and active phase of cervical dilation and effacement and can last from hours to days. Stage 2 is the time from full cervical dilation and effacement to delivery of the fetus and can take minutes to hours. Stage 3 includes the separation and delivery of the placenta and the postdelivery phase and typically lasts between 5 and 30 min (but can last up to an hour) [1]. The length of the first stage of labor typically provides the pregnant patient sufficient time to present to a labor and delivery (L&D) unit. However, various factors can contribute to delays in presentation.

B. Sharp, M.D. (✉)
BerbeeWalsh Department of Emergency Medicine, University of Wisconsin,
800 University Bay Drive, Madison, WI 53705, USA
e-mail: bsharp@medicine.wisc.edu

K. Sharp, M.D.
Department of Obstetrics and Gynecology, University of Wisconsin,
1010 Mound Street, 4th Floor, Madison, WI 53715, USA
e-mail: ksharp2@wisc.edu

E. Wei, M.D., M.B.A.
Department of Emergency Medicine, LAC+USC Medical Center,
2051 Marengo Street, C2K115, Los Angeles, CA 90033, USA
e-mail: EWei@dhs.lacounty.gov

© Springer International Publishing AG 2017
J. Borhart (ed.), *Emergency Department Management of Obstetric Complications*,
DOI 10.1007/978-3-319-54410-6_7

Precipitous labor is defined as delivery of the fetus less than 2–3 h after commencement of regular contractions [1, 2]. Reported rates of precipitous labor vary between 0.07 and 0.6% in the United States [3, 4]. Any ED delivery should be considered and approached as a precipitous delivery. Accelerated or rapid labor and delivery is thought to result from abnormally low resistance of the birth canal, abnormally strong uterine and abdominal contractions, or rarely from the absence of painful sensations. Factors thought to contribute to increased likelihood of precipitous delivery include multiparity, intrauterine growth restriction (IUGR), low birth weight (<2500 g), younger maternal age, lower gestational age, fertility treatments, chronic hypertension, placental abruption, and cocaine use [2–6].

Although the majority of rapid deliveries have good outcomes, rapid labor and delivery can put the mother and fetus at increased risk for complications. These include cervical lacerations, higher-degree perineal lacerations, postpartum hemorrhage, retained placenta, need for blood transfusions, and prolonged hospital stay [5], as well as increased risk of low Apgar scores, admission to the NICU, and mortality when compared to non-precipitous deliveries [4]. Interestingly, attendance of medical personnel at rapid deliveries correlated with no difference in the rate of adverse events [3].

Approach to Precipitous ED Delivery with Normal Fetal Presentation

The vast majority (estimated 95%) of ED deliveries will include normal, cephalic (head first) fetal presentation [1]. It is helpful to consider the following approach when treating these patients.

Preparation

Many EDs have developed a delivery checklist in anticipation of a precipitous or ED delivery. This includes commonly needed equipment that can be prepared and stored in an easily accessible location and will typically consist of adequate lighting, sterile gloves, gown, sterile surgical scissors, two umbilical clamps (or hemostats), bulb suction, dry towels and blankets, diaper, red top tube, radiant warmer/incubator, suction, oxygen (neonatal bag), pediatric and adult code cart/airway management equipment, sterile surgical blades, syringes, needles, and suture material. Of note, continuous fetal heart rate monitoring and uterine activity monitoring should be included, but is typically of limited availability and utility in a precipitous/ED delivery.

Assessment

Obtain as much pregnancy/prenatal history as possible from the mother and/or medical record including gravidity and parity, gestational age, fetal weight, any complications with this pregnancy, and whether rupture of membranes has occurred. It is also helpful to know about outcomes with prior pregnancies (twins, difficult deliveries, cesarean deliveries) and a basic medical history with focus on anything that could complicate resuscitation or lead to potential fetal compromise (i.e., bleeding diathesis or sedating medications/illicit drugs).

A sterile vaginal assessment should be performed, evaluating for any clues that delivery is imminent including a visible fetus emerging (crowning) or any palpable presenting part (arm/leg). If a fluid-filled amniotic sac is visible, take care not to rupture it. Even if a fetus or fetal part is not visible, delivery is likely imminent if the patient is experiencing painful contractions two or less minutes apart, has significant urge to push (reflex if the fetus has descended into the birth canal), and the perineum distends with contractions or you appreciate significant labial separation, anal relaxation/presence of stool, and/or vaginal bleeding. Cervical dilation and effacement should be assessed. Multiparous women will often know the feelings that signal impending birth. If time permits, the presenting part can be determined with bedside ultrasound (i.e., vertex/head down vs. breech), and a fetal heart rate should be obtained via Doppler or auscultation. A normal fetal heart rate is between 110 and 160 bpm with a significant decrease or increase potentially indicating fetal distress. Other important physical exam findings may include maternal fever, which can indicate possible intra-amniotic infection, and hypertension, which can suggest preeclampsia or eclampsia.

The emergency physician must then determine if safe transfer to an obstetric unit can occur. Patients in active labor but not at risk for imminent delivery should be transferred immediately. With fetal presentation at the vaginal outlet (crowning), delivery will need to occur in the ED. If fully effaced and dilated, the patient should probably be delivered in the ED, but will depend on distance and time to L&D unit—i.e., down the hall vs. ambulance ride. Any other scenario will require clinical judgment to determine the best management.

If a patient presents in precipitous labor and with delivery imminent, notify the obstetric provider, the L&D unit, and the pediatrician and/or neonatologist to prepare for any potential complications. This process can be streamlined by use of a birth pager or imminent delivery pager that notifies these appropriate consultants.

Delivery Technique

If it is determined that delivery is imminent, place the mother in the lithotomy position—semi-seated with the hips flexed and abducted and the knees flexed. If no stirrups are available, pillows, towels, or a bedpan should be placed underneath the mother's pelvis to provide additional room to maneuver during delivery. When the mother starts to push, instruct her to tuck her chin to chest and place her hands on the back of her thighs in order to open her pelvis. Rapid breathing or "panting" through the intense portions of contractions and rest with normal breathing between contractions can help to avoid rapid delivery.

During normal delivery, the emergency physician should control the fetus and allow the mother to deliver the baby—not to restrain expulsion. In a normal, vertex (head first) presentation, the fetal head will be engaged at the dilated cervix—typically in a flexed or occiput anterior position with the anterior fontanel toward the posterior perineum. The fetal shoulders then turn obliquely relative to the maternal anterior-posterior (AP) pelvis diameter, allowing passage through the pelvis.

Delivery of the fetal head is facilitated by applying pressure with one hand against the perineum and with the other hand placed on the fetal occiput to control rapid expulsion. Examine the neck for the presence of nuchal cords (umbilical cord wrapped around the neck of the fetus), and if present, attempt reduction by bringing the cord over the fetal head. If the cord is not reducible, it can be left in place or clamped and cut prior to delivery of the shoulders. After delivery of the fetal head, the head will typically rotate to one side (now facing one of the maternal thighs), further turning the shoulder obliquely in the pelvis. Place hands on either side of the fetal head and guide the head gently downward to deliver the anterior shoulder by passing underneath the symphysis pubis. This should be followed with upward traction to deliver the posterior shoulder and body over the perineum. Any difficulty in these maneuvers can be mediated by having an assistant sharply flex the mother's thighs back against her abdomen.

After delivery, perform neonatal resuscitation if necessary, typically starting with suction, drying and stimulating, and more advanced measures as needed. If possible, place the baby on the maternal chest. Early maternal-fetal skin-to-skin contact appears to have benefit on breastfeeding outcomes and infant crying [7]. Place one umbilical clamp or hemostat 10 cm from the fetal abdominal wall with a second 4 cm distal to the first and cut between the clamps with sterile scissors. The clamping does not need to occur urgently but should not be delayed more than 2 min after birth [8]. Collect infant blood in a red top tube to determine newborn's blood type and Rh(D) status.

Delivery of the placenta will typically occur anywhere between 5 and 30 min after delivery of the fetus. There is no reason to hasten what should be a relatively spontaneous process. Clues that placental delivery is occurring include increasingly frequent contractions (that initially slow after delivery), a firm uterus, spontaneous lengthening of the umbilical cord, and a rapid gush of vaginal bleeding. When the placenta begins to protrude from the introitus, grasp the placenta and gently rotate to extract. If the placenta does not deliver with contractions, exert mild traction on the umbilical cord to deliver it while applying pressure on the uterine fundus to avoid uterine inversion. The highest risk for postpartum hemorrhage is typically in the first hour after placental delivery. After placental delivery, apply vigorous uterine pressure with massage to help the uterus contract. If needed, appropriate agents include oxytocin (ideal dose of 20 units in 500 mL crystalloid over 1 h or up to 10 units IM) or methylergonovine. A more detailed discussion of postpartum hemorrhage is contained in Chap. 8 [9–14].

Precipitous/ED Delivery with Abnormal Fetal Presentations

While the vast majority of all deliveries including those in L&D units and in the ED involve normal/cephalic fetal presentation and can be managed with routine delivery care, it is important to be prepared for the rare, but more complicated presentations/deliveries. While incredibly stressful (even to obstetricians), these deliveries can also typically be safely managed with appropriate preparation.

Shoulder Dystocia

Shoulder dystocia is a rare obstetric emergency that occurs in 0.2–3% of live vaginal deliveries [15–17]. Shoulder dystocia is defined as a delivery that requires additional obstetric maneuvers following failure of gentle downward traction on the fetal head to effect delivery of the shoulders or by a prolonged head-to-shoulder delivery interval [18, 19]. This can result from a variety of factors both maternal (small maternal pelvic inlet, inadequate contractions) and fetal (large fetal size, failure of truncal rotation resulting in a transverse instead of oblique orientation of the shoulders). Factors that predict deliveries at risk for a shoulder dystocia include high maternal obesity, maternal diabetes, previous shoulder dystocia, and fetal macrosomia (>4500–5000 g) [19–21]. The correlation between high fetal birth weight and dystocia has been found to be linearly predictive [15], but dystocia can also occur in babies with lower birth weight [20, 21].

Complications

Shoulder dystocia can result in a variety of both maternal and fetal complications. Postpartum hemorrhage (11%) and fourth-degree lacerations (3.8%) are the most commonly reported maternal complications [16, 19, 22]. The risk of fetal injury is as high as 20–40% [19, 23] and includes reported perinatal mortality rates of 0–2.6% [20, 23]. Fetal injuries include brachial plexus palsies (16.8–25%), clavicular fractures (9.5%), humeral fractures (4.2%), and hypoxic-ischemic encephalopathy [19, 23, 24]. Permanent neurologic injury was found to result in up to 13% of cases [20]. Brain injury cases were associated with significantly prolonged head-shoulder times ($\geq$7 min) [25]. However, clinical deterioration can occur out of proportion to the duration of hypoxia due to the combination of compression of the neck leading to central venous congestion and compression of the umbilical cord reducing placental flow produce as well as decreased uterine blood flow after delivery of the fetal head [26].

Technique

Shoulder dystocia can be heralded by delivery of fetal head with subsequent retraction after attempt at downward traction (i.e., the turtle sign), indicating that typically the anterior shoulder is impacted on the pubic bone. There are two helpful mnemonics that can be applied to remember a systematic approach to shoulder dystocia. They are HELPERR and ALARMER (Table 7.1).

The first step in approaching a shoulder dystocia is to call for help. Even more assistance is often needed than would be required in a typical precipitous delivery. This will become important in the various maneuvers described. There is also greater potential for fetal injury and need for fetal resuscitation.

The first or primary maneuvers in a shoulder dystocia are McRoberts maneuver and suprapubic pressure. These have the highest chance of success and the lowest risk of fetal injury. These two maneuvers move the maternal pubic symphysis more cephalad and typically release the anterior shoulder. McRoberts maneuver requires two assistants—each one holding a leg with the knees and hips flexed and the thighs held against the abdomen (Fig. 7.1). McRoberts maneuver has been shown by x-ray not to increase the pelvic diameter but rather to facilitate cephalad rotation of the symphysis pubis with flattening/straightening of the sacrum [27]. This allows the posterior shoulder to be pushed over the sacral promontory and fall into the hollow of the sacrum, while the symphysis rotates over the impacted anterior shoulder.

One assistant should apply suprapubic pressure with the heel of their hand just over the mother's pubic bone and over the anterior fetal shoulder. Downward and lateral pressure applied to the posterior aspect of the impacted, anterior fetal shoulder should facilitate adduction of the anterior shoulder, decreasing the fetal diameter and allowing for passage of the anterior shoulder under the symphysis pubis. Initially

Table 7.1 Mnemonics for shoulder dystocia

HELPERR	
H	Call for help
E	Evaluate for episiotomy
L	Legs (McRobert's Maneuver by assistant)
P	Suprapubic pressure (by assistant)
E	Enter maneuvers/internal rotation (Rubin's, Woods Corkscrew)
R	Remove posterior arm
R	Roll the patient (Gaskin Manuever)
ALARMER	
A	Ask for help
L	Leg hyperflexion (McRoberts)
A	Anterior shoulder disimpaction (suprapubic pressure)
R	Rotational maneuvers (Rubin II, Woods Corkscrew)
M	Manual delivery of posterior arm
E	Evaluate for episiotomy
R	Roll the patient (Gaskin)

Fig. 7.1 McRoberts
maneuver performed with
two assistants. Assistant on
patient's left applies
suprapubic pressure. Image
courtesy CAE Healthcare,
with permission

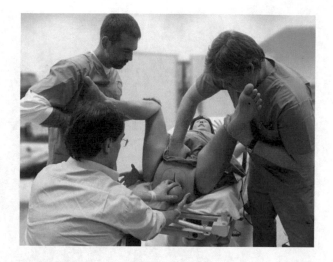

continuous, the pressure can also be applied in a rocking motion similar to chest compressions. Fundal pressure should never be applied as it only worsens impaction on the pelvic brim, potentially injuring the fetus or mother [28]. McRoberts alone has been shown to be successful between 40 and 58% of the time [22, 29, 30]. When suprapubic pressure is added, success rates of 54 and 58% have been found [22, 29].

If primary maneuvers (McRoberts and suprapubic pressure) are unsuccessful, secondary maneuvers to consider include rotational maneuvers or delivery of the posterior arm. These are necessary in approximately 1/3 of cases [31]. Although typically signifying a greater degree of dystocia, these maneuvers are not actually associated with a higher risk of maternal or fetal injury [19, 32]. An episiotomy should be considered, but not routinely performed when a shoulder dystocia is encountered. An episiotomy will not in itself alleviate the primary problem in a shoulder dystocia (a bone on bone impaction), and prophylactic episiotomy with delivery does not reduce the risk of shoulder dystocia occurring [33]. Episiotomy has also been associated with a sevenfold increase in the rate of severe perineal trauma [34]. However, episiotomy does provide additional space for the physician's hand to successfully perform the various internal maneuvers to alleviate the shoulder dystocia. With the high success rate of McRoberts maneuver and suprapubic pressure, it is most appropriate to wait until additional maneuvers are required before performing an episiotomy.

The focus of internal rotation maneuvers is to allow entry of the fetal shoulders into the pelvic inlet in a transverse or oblique diameter. The most popular internal rotation maneuvers include the Rubin II maneuver and Woods corkscrew maneuver. Rubin II maneuver involves placement of fingers behind the posterior aspect of the anterior shoulder of the fetus and rotating the shoulder toward the fetal chest (Fig. 7.2). The resulting adduction of the fetal shoulder girdle reduces the shoulders' diameter, potentially alleviating the dystocia. Woods corkscrew maneuver involves continued application of the pressure on the anterior shoulder (as in Rubin II), with additional upward pressure placed on the anterior aspect of the fetal posterior shoulder toward the fetal back, leading to posterior shoulder abduction

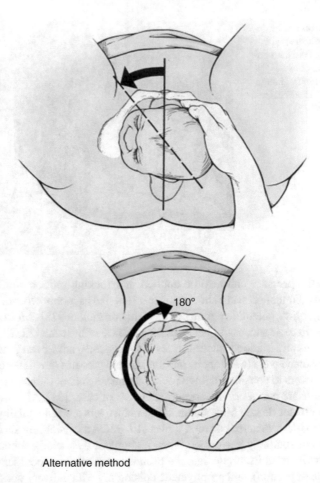

Alternative method

Fig. 7.2 Rubin II rotation of the anterior shoulder forward into the fetal chest (*top*). Reverse Woods corkscrew place fingers behind posterior shoulder and rotate fetus in the opposite direction of Rubin II (*bottom*). From Gabbe SG, eds. *Obstetrics: Normal and Problem Pregnancies.* Philadelphia: Churchill Livingstone, 2017; *with permission*

(Fig. 7.2). This creates additive force in the same circumferential arc as Rubin II, resulting in more effective rotation. The McRoberts maneuver also can be applied during this maneuver and may facilitate its success. If the Rubin II or Woods corkscrew maneuvers fail, the reverse Woods corkscrew maneuver may be tried. In this maneuver, the physician's fingers are placed on the back of the posterior shoulder of the fetus, and the fetus is rotated in the opposite direction as in the Woods corkscrew or Rubin II maneuvers.

If internal rotation maneuvers fail, delivery of the posterior arm should be considered. Place a hand behind the posterior fetal shoulder, tracing the arm to the elbow, where pressure is applied to the antecubital fossa to flex the fetal forearm

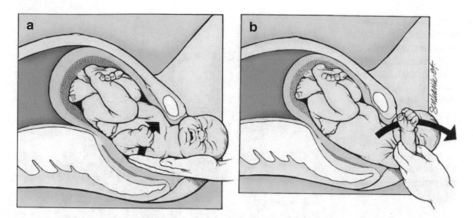

Fig. 7.3 Delivery of the posterior arm. The operator here inserts a hand (a) and sweeps the posterior arm across the chest and over the perineum (b). Care should be taken to distribute the pressure evenly across the humerus to avoid unnecessary fracture. From Gabbe SG, eds. *Obstetrics: Normal and Problem Pregnancies*. Philadelphia: Churchill Livingstone, 2017; *with permission*

(Fig. 7.3). The arm is then swept out over the fetal chest and delivered. Often, the fetus follows with spontaneous rotation after the arm is removed, leading to alleviation of impaction of the anterior shoulder. Grasping or pulling of the arm or pressure directly on the humeral shaft should be avoided. This maneuver is associated with an increased rate of humeral fracture.

Rotational maneuvers were not associated with a higher fetal injury risk compared with McRoberts maneuver [35]. Individual maneuvers (Rubin, Woods screw, delivery of posterior arm) were not associated with increased composite morbidity, neonatal injury, or neonatal depression after adjusting for nulliparity and duration of shoulder dystocia.

The next maneuver to consider is to roll the patient into an "all fours" position—referred to as the Gaskin maneuver (Fig. 7.4). This has been demonstrated to increase obstetric conjugate by as much as 10 mm with pelvic outlet increasing by as much as 10 mm [36]. This increased space with the addition of gravity is often enough to deliver the posterior shoulder and arm and allow for disimpaction of the anterior shoulder from the pubic symphysis. Gaskin maneuver was found to be successful in over 80% of women who required progression to this maneuver [37]. Internal maneuvers may be repeated while the patient is on "all fours" if simply moving into this position does not result in delivery.

Heroic maneuvers should be considered only after all other maneuvers have failed. These include cephalic replacement (Zavanelli) followed by cesarean section, symphysiotomy (used more widely in developing countries), deliberate clavicular fracture (to reduce bisacromial diameter), hysterotomy (to allow rotation from intrauterine pressure), and delivery under general anesthesia.

Fig. 7.4 The Gaskin position. The "all fours" position exploits the effects of gravity and increased space in the hollow of the sacrum to facilitate delivery of the posterior shoulder and arm. From Gottlieb AG, Galan HL. Shoulder dystocia: An update. Obstet Gynecol Clin N Am. 2007;34:501–531; with permission

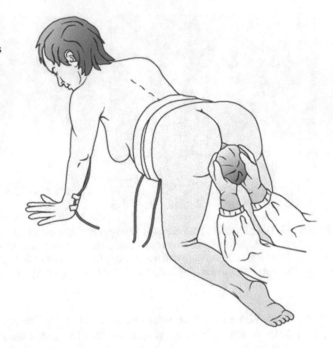

Management of Umbilical Cord Prolapse

Umbilical cord prolapse occurs when all or part of the umbilical cord precedes the fetal presenting part. This is associated with abnormal presentations, situations where the presenting part does not fill the entire cervical canal, or with a long umbilical cord. Resulting compression of the umbilical cord can result in fetal hypoxia, distress, and asphyxiation.

With an umbilical cord prolapse and a viable fetus, cesarean delivery is the method of delivery of choice. Maneuvers to preserve circulation should be instituted immediately. Attempt should be made to digitally elevate the presenting part from the umbilical cord and place the mother in Trendelenburg or in an "all fours" position. Advise the patient not to push. Placement of a Foley catheter and instilling 500 mL saline may help lift the fetus off the cord. Preparation for emergency cesarean should be underway. Manipulation and cord trauma should be kept to a minimum. If there is no option for surgical management, the umbilical cord may be pushed gently in a retrograde fashion above the presenting part. Subsequent to delivery, the physician should be prepared for resuscitation of a distressed infant.

Management of Breech Delivery

Breech presentation is the presentation of fetal feet or buttocks. It is an obstetric emergency that occurs in 3–4% of term pregnancies [38, 39] with a higher incidence in preterm deliveries (due to the fact that final natural fetal rotation may not yet have

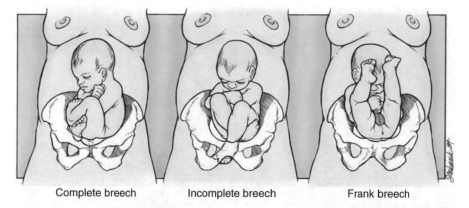

Complete breech   Incomplete breech   Frank breech

Fig. 7.5 The *complete breech* is flexed at the hips and flexed at the knees. The *incomplete breech* shows incomplete flexion of one or both knees or hips. The *frank breech* is flexed at the hips and extended at the knees. From Gabbe SG, eds. *Obstetrics: Normal and Problem Pregnancies.* Philadelphia: Churchill Livingstone, 2017; *with permission*

occurred) and with advanced maternal age [40]. Breech presentation is associated with a morbidity rate 3–4 times greater than that of normal cephalic presentations [38]. It increases the likelihood of umbilical cord prolapse and dystocia during delivery. During a normal delivery, the head, which is larger than the buttocks, maximally dilates the cervix with the body following, while in a breech delivery, the buttock does not adequately dilate the cervix to allow for passage of the diameter of the head. A dystocia can then occur after delivery of the buttock and body as the head is stuck with resultant umbilical cord compression, fractures, spinal cord injuries, and potential asphyxiation and fetal death as delivery of the head is attempted.

There are three types of breech presentation. In the ED, they are all associated with high rates of dystocia and poor fetal outcomes, especially for full-term infants. Types include frank breech (buttocks first with knees extended and feet adjacent to the head), which represents 65–70% of breech deliveries; complete (buttocks first with knees/hips flexed, i.e., cross-legged); and incomplete/footling (one or both feet below—rare) (Fig. 7.5).

If a breech presentation is recognized on initial cervical examination or bedside ultrasound, the patient should be moved to L&D if at all possible to facilitate a cesarean delivery. If transfer is not possible, call for help immediately including obstetric and pediatric colleagues. Premature infants in the breech often deliver spontaneously likely secondary to their small size, but as the infant gets closer to term, dystocia will be more common. Care should be taken to avoid iatrogenic rupture of membranes as this can lead to umbilical cord prolapse. Try to delay maternal pushing to allow for the arrival of an obstetrician.

If delay is not possible, then an assisted breech delivery will be required (Fig. 7.6). The patient should be placed in the lithotomy position. Evaluate for umbilical cord prolapse. Encourage the mother to bear down until the feet/leg and then trunk are visible. Support the fetal body outside of the birth canal but do not elevate or apply any traction as delivery progresses. Do not pull on the breech. Allow for spontaneous

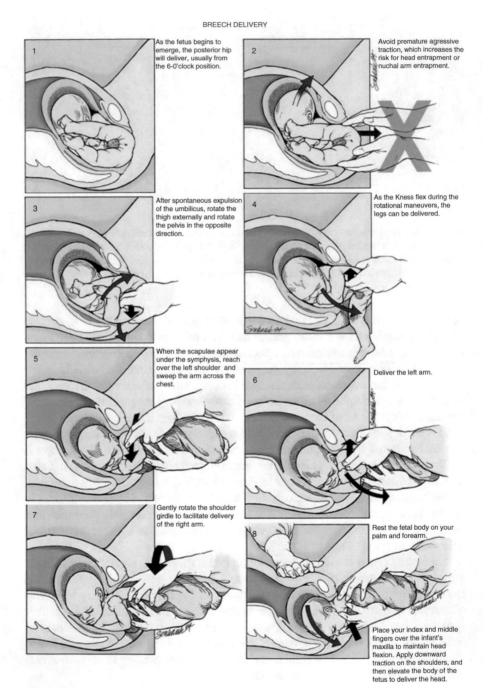

BREECH DELIVERY

1 As the fetus begins to emerge, the posterior hip will deliver, usually from the 6-0'clock position.

2 Avoid premature agressive traction, which increases the risk for head entrapment or nuchal arm entrapment.

3 After spontaneous expulsion of the umbilicus, rotate the thigh externally and rotate the pelvis in the opposite direction.

4 As the Kness flex during the rotational maneuvers, the legs can be delivered.

5 When the scapulae appear under the symphysis, reach over the left shoulder and sweep the arm across the chest.

6 Deliver the left arm.

7 Gently rotate the shoulder girdle to facilitate delivery of the right arm.

8 Rest the fetal body on your palm and forearm.

Place your index and middle fingers over the infant's maxilla to maintain head flexion. Apply downward traction on the shoulders, and then elevate the body of the fetus to deliver the head.

Fig. 7.6 Breech delivery. From: Roberts JR, eds. Clinical Procedures in Emergency Medicine. Philadelphia: Elsevier Saunders, 2014; with permission

Table 7.2 Management of vaginal breech delivery	Explain necessity of effective pushing in the second stage of labor
	Adequate maternal analgesia
	Spontaneous descent and expulsion to the umbilicus with maternal pushing ONLY
	Do not pull on the breech
	Rotation to sacrum anterior is desired and can be facilitated
	Do not attempt to extract the legs
	If needed can assist by flexing leg at the hips once popliteal fossa is visible
	Do not hold by the abdomen
	May rotate body to facilitate delivery of the arms over the chest
	Support to maintain head in flexed position
	Maternal expulsive efforts should be encouraged

delivery until the umbilicus is visualized. The fetal pelvis (not abdomen) should be grasped by using a sterile towel and delivered until the scapula is visualized. The neonate should be kept in a sacrum anterior position. If the arms do not deliver at this point, the infant should be rotated 90° to allow for delivery of the arms. If this does not occur spontaneously, place a finger into the antecubital fossa to facilitate delivery of each arm. Another rotation of 180° may now be needed to deliver the posterior shoulder. Delivery of the head should occur with the fetus against the sacrum anterior [41]. The Mauriceau-Smellie-Veit maneuver involves use of index and middle finger to put pressure on the fetal maxilla to flex the fetal neck. Excessive upward angulation and traction can cause neck hyperextension with cervical spinal cord injury. If the head cannot be delivered quickly, poor fetal outcome is anticipated. If this occurs, one can consider uterine relaxants such as terbutaline or nitroglycerine. Table 7.2 reviews management guidelines for breech delivery if this is encountered in the ED.

Summary

Precipitous delivery is a stressful event. Emergency physicians can prepare for ED deliveries by developing delivery checklists, kits, and appropriate expedited consultant notification (i.e., paging lists). The majority of precipitous deliveries will result in good outcomes for mother and baby, but emergency physicians must be prepared to manage the various complications. Management of shoulder dystocia should begin with McRoberts maneuver and application of suprapubic pressure and proceed to rotational or internal maneuvers. In the case of prolapsed umbilical cord, elevate the presenting fetal part to alleviate pressure on the cord and obtain obstetric assistance for emergent cesarean section. Breech delivery is best managed by allowing the mother to deliver the fetus with no assistance in delivery until the umbilicus is visualized.

Key Points

- Most precipitous deliveries will result in good outcomes for mother and baby with adequate preparation.
- Have an ED birth or imminent delivery paging list set up and a supply checklist in your ED.
- For shoulder dystocia, start with the McRoberts maneuver and be prepared to progress to subsequent maneuvers.
- Never apply fundal pressure in a shoulder dystocia.
- If a prolapsed cord is identified, first elevate the presenting fetal part.
- In a breech delivery, touch the fetus only when you see the umbilicus, and never pull on the fetus.

References

1. Kilpatrick S, Garrison E. Normal labor and delivery. In: Obstetrics: normal and problem pregnancies. Philadelphia, PA: Churchill Livingston; 2007. p. 303–21.
2. Suzuki S. Clinical significance of precipitous labor. J Clin Med Res. 2015;7:150–3.
3. Sheiner E, Hershkovitz R, Shoham I, Erez O, Hadar A, Mazor M. A retrospective study of unplanned out-of-hospital deliveries. Arch Gynecol Obstet. 2004;269:85–8.
4. Rodie V, Thomson A, Norman J. Accidental out-of-hospital deliveries: an obstetric and neonatal case control study. Acta Obstet Gynecol Scand. 2002;81:50–4.
5. Sheiner E, Levy A, Mazor M. Precipitate labor: higher rates of maternal complications. Eur J Obstet Gynecol Reprod Biol. 2004;116(1):43–7.
6. Mahon TR, Chazotte C, Cohen WR. Short labor: characteristics and outcome. Obstet Gynecol. 1994;84(1):47–51.
7. Anderson GC, Moore E, Hepworth J, Bergman N. Early skin-to-skin contact for mothers and their healthy newborn infants. Cochrane Database Syst Rev. 2003;(2). Art. No.: CD003519. Doi: 10.1002/14651858.CD003519.
8. Hutton EK, Hassan ES. Late vs early clamping of the umbilical cord in full-term neonates: systematic review and meta-analysis of controlled trials. JAMA. 2007;297(11):1241–52.
9. McBee P, Burnie G. ED precipitous labor and delivery flow sheet. J Emerg Nurs. 1995;21:326–8.
10. Robinson L. Preparing for precipitous vaginal deliveries in the Emergency Department. J Emerg Nurs. 2009;35(3):256–9.
11. Schorn M, Wilbeck J. Unexpected birth in the emergency department: the role of the advanced practice nurse. Adv Emerg Nurs J. 2009;31(2):170–7.
12. Silver D, Sabatino F. Precipitous and difficult deliveries. Emerg Med Clin N Am. 2012;30:961–75.
13. Soremekun O. Pregnancy, precipitous delivery. Encyclopedia Intensive Care Med. 1815–1819.
14. Blake C. "Did you just say. The Baby's Coming!!?" A Nurse's guide to prepare for a safe precipitous delivery in the emergency department. J Emerg Nurs. 2012;38(3):296–300.
15. Gherman R, Chauhan S, Ouzounian J, Lerner H, et al. Shoulder dystocia: the unpreventable obstetric emergency with empiric management guidelines. Am J Obstet Gynecol. 2006;195:657–72.
16. Hoffman M, Bailit J, Branch DW, Burkman R, Veldhusien P, Lu L, Kominiarek M, et al. A comparison of obstetric maneuvers for the acute management of shoulder dystocia. Obstet Gynecol. 2011;117(6):1272–8.

17. Kwek K, Yeo G. Shoulder dystocia and injuries: prevention and management. Curr Opin Obstet Gynecol. 2006;18:123–8.
18. American College of Obstetrics and Gynecologists. Shoulder dystocia. ACOG Practice bulletin no. 40. Obstet Gynecol. 2002;100:1045–50.
19. Gherman R, Ouzounian J, Goodwin T. Obstetric maneuvers for shoulder dystocia and associated fetal morbidity. Am J Obstet Gynecol. 1997;178(6):1126–30.
20. Beall M, Spong C, McKay J, Ross M. Objective definition of shoulder dystocia: a prospective evaluation. Am J Obstet Gynecol. 1998;179(4):934–7.
21. Geary M, McParland P, Johnson H, Stronge J. Shoulder dystocia—is it predictable? Eur J Obstet Gynecol. 1995;62:15–8.
22. Gherman R, Goodwin TM, Souter I, Neumann K, Ouzounian J, Paul R. The McRoberts' maneuver for the alleviation of shoulder dystocia: how successful is it? Am J Obstet Gynecol. 1996;176(3):656–61.
23. Christoffersson M, Rydhstroem H. Shoulder dystocia and brachial plexus injury: a population-based study. Gynecol Obstet Invest. 2002;53(1):42–7.
24. Chauhan SP, Rose CH, Gherman RB, Magann EF, Holland MW, Morrison JC. Brachial plexus injury: a 23-year experience from a tertiary center. Am J Obstet Gynecol. 2005;192(6):1795–800.
25. Ouzounian JG, Korst LM, Ahn MO, et al. Shoulder dystocia and neonatal brain injury: significant of the head-sholder interval. Am J Obstet Gynecol. 1998;178:S76.
26. Baskett T. Shoulder dystocia. Best Pract Res Clin Obstet Gynaecol. 2002;16(1):57–68.
27. Gherman RB, Tramont J, Muffley P, et al. Analysis of McRoberts' maneuver by X-ray pelvimetry. Obstet Gynecol. 2000;95:43–7.
28. Gross SJ, Shime J, Farine D. Shoulder dystocia: predictors and outcome. Am J Obstet Gynecol. 1987;156:334–6.
29. Macfarland MB, Langer O, Piper JM, Berkus MD. Perinatal outcome and the type and number of maneuvers in shoulder dystocia. Int J Gynaecol Obstet. 1996;55:219–24.
30. Spain J, Frey H, Tuuli M, Colvin R, Macones G, Cahill A. Neonatal morbidity associated with shoulder dystocia maneuvers. Am J Obstet Gynecol. 2015;353:e1–5.
31. Stallings SP, Edwards RK, Johnson JWC. Correlation of head-to-body delivery intervals in shoulder dystocia and umbilical artery acidosis. Am J Obstet Gynecol. 2001;185:268–74.
32. Gherman R. Shoulder dystocia: an evidence-based evaluation of the obstetric nightmare. Clin Obstet Gynecol. 2002;45(2):345–62.
33. Youssef R, Ramalingam U, Macleod M, et al. Cohort study of maternal and neonatal morbidity in relation to use of episiotomy at instrumental vaginal delivery. BJOG. 2005;112:941–5.
34. Gurewitsch ED, Donithan M, Stallings SP, Moore PL, Agarwal S, Allen LM, et al. Episiotomy versus fetal manipulation in managing severe shoulder dystocia: a comparison of outcomes. Am J Obstet Gynecol. 2004;191:911–6.
35. Leung T, Stuart O, Suen SSSH, Sahota DS, Lau TK, Lao TT. Comparison of perinatal outcomes of shoulder dystocia alleviated by different type and sequence of manoeuvres: a retrospective review. BJOG. 2011;118:985–90.
36. Baxley E, Gobbo R. Shoulder dystocia. Am Fam Physician. 2004;6917:1707–14.
37. Bruner J, Drummond S, Meenan A, et al. All-fours maneuver for reducing shoulder dystocia during labor. J Reprod Med. 1998;43(5):439–43.
38. Hearne A, Driggers R. The Johns Hopkins manual of gynecology and obstetrics. 2nd ed. Baltimore, MD: Johns Hopkins University Press; 2002.
39. Martin JA, Hamilton BE, Sutton PD, Ventura SJ, Menacker F, Munson ML. Births: final data for 2002. Natl Vital Stat Rep. 2003;52(10):1–113.
40. Brown L, Karrison T, Cibilis L. Mode of delivery and perinatal results in breech presentation. AJOG. 1994;171(1):28–34.
41. Susan M, Seeds M, Seeds J. Malpresentation. In: Obstetrics: normal and problem pregnancies. Philadelphia, PA: Churchill Livingston; p. 428–55.

Chapter 8
Evaluation and Treatment of Postpartum Hemorrhage

Elaine Bromberek and Janet Smereck

Introduction

Severe uterine bleeding after childbirth presents a major life threat for the patient and unique management challenges for the emergency physician. Postpartum hemorrhage (PPH) is a significant cause of morbidity and mortality, leading to over 150,000 deaths per year on average worldwide. It is reported as the third leading cause of maternal mortality in the USA, complicating as many as 15% of deliveries [1–7]. Initial steps in the emergency department (ED) management of the patient with PPH involve estimation of the quantity of blood loss and identification of the probable underlying cause to determine urgency and guide appropriate therapeutic interventions.

Postpartum hemorrhage has various definitions in the literature. One definition is blood loss in excess of 500 ml after vaginal delivery and 1000 ml after cesarean delivery, with blood loss in excess of 1000 ml constituting severe PPH [5, 8, 9]. PPH is further divided into two categories: primary PPH and secondary PPH. Primary PPH is defined as excess bleeding which occurs in the first 24 h after delivery. As such, primary PPH is most likely to be managed in the obstetrical ward, although home births and precipitous deliveries may bring this complication to the ED. The American College of Obstetricians and Gynecologists (ACOG) specifies severe primary PPH as blood loss greater than 1000 ml within 24 h following the birth process accompanied by signs and symptoms of hypovolemia [10]. Secondary PPH, defined as any abnormal vaginal bleeding occurring after 24 h up to 6 weeks after delivery,

E. Bromberek, M.D. (✉)
Department of Emergency Medicine, MedStar Georgetown University and MedStar Washington Hospital Center, 110 Irving St NW, Washington, DC 20010, USA
e-mail: elaine.f.bromberek@medstar.net

J. Smereck, M.D.
Department of Emergency Medicine, MedStar Georgetown University Hospital, Washington, DC, USA
e-mail: janet.a.smereck@medstar.net

© Springer International Publishing AG 2017
J. Borhart (ed.), *Emergency Department Management of Obstetric Complications*,
DOI 10.1007/978-3-319-54410-6_8

is less common, complicating 0.5–15% of deliveries [3, 11, 12]. The quantity of blood loss in secondary PPH is more subjective and generally is defined as bleeding sufficient to require emergency management, including blood transfusion [12].

The various definitions of PPH often invoke imprecise measures including visual estimates of blood loss and pad counts [8, 13–15]. Visual estimates tend to underestimate and under-recognize large-volume hemorrhage [14, 16]. A more practical clinical definition of severe PPH is postpartum bleeding necessitating emergency treatment modalities including blood transfusions, surgical repair, uterine artery embolization, and hysterectomy [17]. The shock index, defined as the ratio of pulse to systolic blood pressure, has been evaluated for obstetrical hemorrhage. An index greater than 0.9–1.1 correlates with severe PPH and the need for therapeutic interventions such as blood transfusion [18–21] (Fig. 8.1).

Risk Factors for Severe Postpartum Hemorrhage

Knowing which patients who are at increased risk for severe PPH can lead to proactive management and improved outcomes (Table 8.1). Prolonged labor and previous cesarean delivery strongly predict severe blood loss in women with PPH [3]. Both the presence of uterine fibroids and a history of treatment for fibroids, either by myomectomy or uterine artery embolization, are associated with increased risk [12, 22]. A prolonged third stage of labor (>20 min) specifically predisposes patients to severe PPH. Active management of placental delivery, including uterotonic drug administration, fundal massage, and controlled cord traction, may decrease the duration of the third stage of labor, thus decreasing the risk of hemorrhage [23].

Etiologies of Primary Postpartum Hemorrhage

Uterine atony, the failure of the uterus to contract following labor, is the most common cause of primary PPH [7, 24]. Risk factors for uterine atony include conditions causing overdistention of the uterus such as multiple birth pregnancy and fetal macrosomia, prolonged labor, and deep anesthetic use [25–27]. Maternal obesity (body mass index 40 or higher) increases the risk of atonic uterine hemorrhage [28]. Although breast-feeding may have a uterotonic effect due to endogenous oxytocin, this does not necessarily prevent PPH due to uterine atony [24].

An atonic uterus is "boggy" from the failure of myometrial fibers to contract. It is palpable on bimanual exam as softer than a typical, contracted post-delivery uterus. Initial management consists of bimanual uterine massage, which stimulates myometrial fibers to contract. Bimanual massage involves forceful compression of the uterus, with one hand providing external pressure on the lower abdomen and the other hand providing intravaginal pressure on the cervix [26] (Fig. 8.2). Bimanual compression is more effective when performed by a two-person team. One provider

Case Example

A 36–year–old female, Gravida 1 Para 1, presented to the ED 5 days after normal spontaneous vaginal delivery (NSVD) with sudden onset of heavy vaginal bleeding, rapidly soaking large several towels with dark red blood in a 30–min interval. She reported pelvic cramping and light–headedness on arrival to the ED. Delivery was at term and uncomplicated, with estimated blood loss of 400 cc and an intact placenta noted in obstetrical records. Lochia was scanty in the interval following discharge from the hospital the day following delivery until presentation to the ED. The patient had no history of menorrhagia or coagulopathy; her infant was healthy and reported to be breast-feeding well.

On examination, the patient appeared pale and anxious with an initial heart rate of 133 beats per minute and blood pressure 109/61; she was afebrile. Pertinent physical findings included mild suprapubic tenderness, with a firm uterine fundus palpable above the pubic rim; vaginal examination revealed active bleeding with large clots of blood in the vagina.

Initial management included placement of two large bore peripheral intravenous (IV) lines and infusion of normal saline, 2 l by rapid bolus. Blood was obtained for complete blood count (CBC) and type and screen. Heart rate response to crystalloid infusion was initially favorable; heart rate fell to the 70s and blood pressure was unchanged; the patient reported feeling less dizzy. Initial hematocrit returned at 36.8 with hemoglobin 12.7 and platelet count 309 × 103. The on-call obstetrician was consulted but not immediately available to examine the patient; oxytocin for intravenous infusion was requested from the pharmacy. The emergency physician performed bimanual compression; the uterine fundus was felt to be firm, and compression of the cervix was suboptimal due to the presence of large blood clots. Ultrasound examination at the bedside revealed hemorrhage within the endometrial cavity with open internal and external os and a large hematoma within the endocervical canal. There was no sonographic evidence for retained products of conception.

A sudden increase in observed vaginal bleeding then occurred. Blood pressure fell to 85/57 and heart rate increased to 112 beats per minute. Hemoglobin fell to 9.6 and hematocrit fell to 27.9 on recheck. Uncrossmatched O negative blood was ordered for transfusion, and central venous access was obtained. Oxytocin infusion was initiated. Vaginal bleeding continued at a brisk rate and blood pressure fell as low as 54/28; the patient became pale and less responsive. Methylergonovine injection and oral misoprostol were ordered, and interventional radiology was consulted for potential uterine artery embolization to assist in hemorrhage control.

Blood was rapidly transfused and a third unit was ordered. The obstetric team examined the patient in the ED and confirmed the presence of a firm uterine fundus. Two obstetric providers performed a speculum examination and evacuated a 12 cm by 3 cm clot from the cervix. No cervical or vaginal lacerations were detected, and the hemorrhage ceased after clot extraction allowed for vigorous two-person manual compression to achieve effective contraction of the lower uterine segment and cervix.

Following endocervical clot extraction, administration of uterotonic medications, and infusions of a total of 4 l of crystalloid and three units of packed red blood cells, the patient's blood pressure rose to 119/52 and her level of alertness improved. She was observed in the hospital without further hemorrhage or need for invasive intervention and discharged after a period of observation, in stable condition.

Fig. 8.1 The above case, a patient presenting to the ED with severe secondary PPH, illustrates some of the unique management challenges requiring coordinated efforts across departments in order to optimize care

Table 8.1 Factors
predisposing to postpartum
hemorrhage

• Pregnancy with multiple fetuses
• Fetal macrosomia
• Fetal malpresentation
• Prior uterine incision or myomectomy
• Prolonged labor
• Prolonged third stage (>20 min)
• Previous postpartum hemorrhage
• Placenta previa
• Maternal obesity (BMI > 40)
• Inherited coagulopathy

Fig. 8.2 Bimanual uterine
massage. Francois KE,
Foley MR. Antepartum
and postpartum
hemorrhage. *Obstetrics:
Normal and Problem
Pregnancies.* Ed. Steven
G. Gabbe. Philadelphia:
Elsevier, 2016. 407. Print.
With permission

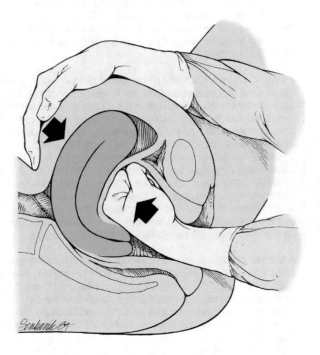

maintains external pressure to the uterine fundus, while a second provider places
pressure on the lower uterine segment. This technique allows for sustained duration
of compression, which may be required to achieve effective uterine contraction [29].

Traumatic lacerations to the vagina and cervix during delivery are another cause
of PPH. Direct visualization of the vaginal walls and cervix is required for diagnosis
and repair. Although ongoing hemorrhage will likely obscure a clear view, all possible efforts should be made for direct inspection after uterine atony has been
excluded and treated by examination and bimanual compression [7].

Placenta that is partially or completely retained can cause hemorrhage shortly
after delivery. Examination of the placenta after delivery is necessary to ensure it is
complete, without any missing segments that may remain in the uterus. Retained
placenta must be removed for bleeding to stop. Manual removal is achieved by
sweeping the uterus digitally or with surgical instruments; mechanical evacuation of
retained placenta is more effective than pharmacologic maneuvers [30, 31].

Table 8.2 Etiologies of postpartum hemorrhage

Primary hemorrhage:	Secondary hemorrhage:
• Uterine atony	• Uterine atony
• Traumatic lacerations	• Subinvolution of placental site
• Retained placenta	• Retained products of conception
• Abnormal placentation	• Retained placenta
• Placenta accrete	• Endometritis
• Coagulopathy	• Coagulopathy
• DIC	• DIC
• TTP	• Uterine artery pseudoaneurysm
• ITP	
• HELLP	
• Von Willebrand disease	
• Thrombocytopenia	
• Hemophilia carrier	
• Uterine inversion	

Abnormal placental implantation can also contribute to PPH [9, 32]. In the case of placenta accreta, the placenta invades the myometrium and incompletely separates at birth, leading to open sinuses, which predispose to severe hemorrhage [32]. Placenta accreta is subclassified into placenta increta or placenta percreta, based on involvement of placenta into or through the myometrium [27]. When retained products are due to placenta accreta, PPH can be especially difficult to control and hysterectomy is often necessary. Risk factors for placenta accreta include prior placenta previa and prior invasive gynecologic and obstetric procedures including uterine incisions, endometrial ablation, and uterine artery embolization [22].

Uterine inversion is a life-threatening but rare obstetric complication that can lead to postpartum hemorrhage. It is identified by visualization or palpation of the uterine fundus in the introitus or vaginal vault and by the inability to palpate the uterine fundus in the abdomen. Associated shock syndrome is due to blood loss, with some component of parasympathetic response to excessive traction on the malpositioned uterus [32–34]. The severe degree of shock may appear out of proportion to visualized blood loss. Incomplete inversion can occur with a more occult presentation, in which the fundus inverts but remains within the body of the uterus [33]. Ultrasound is helpful in confirming the diagnosis if it is unclear based on physical exam alone. Ultrasound may show an "inside out" or "upside down" sign, with the fundus displaced toward the vagina or in the uterine body [35]. Although often attributed to adherent placenta or excessive cord traction, the cause of uterine inversion is often unknown. Table 8.2 summarizes the commonly reported etiologies of primary PPH.

Etiologies of Secondary Postpartum Hemorrhage

Secondary postpartum hemorrhage occurs in approximately 1% of pregnancies, and many identifiable causes overlap with those implicated in primary PPH. However, in one study spanning 9 years, no cause was determined in 16.7% of cases of secondary PPH, and when determined, the diagnosis was most often based on histopathologic findings. As with primary PPH, uterine atony, retained products of conception, subinvolution of the placental site, and coagulopathies are the etiologies most often identified [36] (Table 8.2).

Retained products of conception (POC) commonly present as a cause of secondary PPH. Persistence of the trophoblastic villi and increased vascularity to retained POC are sources of hemorrhage. Retained placenta can also lead to subinvolution of the placental site and uterine atony, leading to multifaceted causes for hemorrhage. Ultrasound imaging may show a thickened endometrium or intrauterine mass with vascular color flow on Doppler [37].

Placental site subinvolution is the failure of uteroplacental vessels to close after delivery. Normally after delivery, placental vessels involute to constrict the dilated uteroplacental vessels caused by normal pregnancy physiology. In the case of subinvolution, arteries remain dilated when they should be closing, which can lead to massive blood loss postpartum [38]. Subinvolution was found as the cause of 13.3% of cases of secondary postpartum hemorrhage in one report. It is often associated with retained products of conception [36]. A diagnosis can be suggested by ultrasound showing increased myometrial vascularity and low resistance flow, which can appear similar to retained POC or arteriovenous malformation [39].

Endometritis, an infection of the endometrium after delivery by a combination of aerobes and anaerobes, is another causative factor in secondary PPH [36]. Characterized by fever, pelvic pain, and uterine tenderness with or without purulent lochia, endometritis can rapidly progress to toxic shock syndrome, sepsis, or necrotizing myometritis. Postpartum infections also predispose the patient to hemorrhage due to acquired coagulopathies. Release of cytokines associated with severe infection leads to activation of the fibrinolytic system and the coagulation cascade, which can quickly progress to disseminated intravascular coagulation (DIC). Specifically, a few cases have been reported of endometritis due to *Clostridium* bacteria, which release a hemorrhagic toxin leading to toxic shock syndrome [40]. Hemodynamic instability can occur with hemorrhagic and septic shock occurring simultaneously. Treatment should include broad-spectrum antibiotic coverage of anaerobic and gram-negative bacteria [41].

Uterine artery pseudoaneurysm, a rare cause of secondary PPH, is a collection of blood that communicates with arterial blood flow. It is usually associated with cesarean delivery, as there is potential for trauma to the uterine artery. Pseudoaneurysm occurs when a hematoma forms around leakage from the uterine artery and a communication persists. Hemorrhage can be intra-abdominal or vaginal depending on the location of the hematoma [42]. Alternatively, the pseudoaneurysm can rupture, leading to sudden and potentially massive blood loss [43].

Hematologic Considerations in Postpartum Hemorrhage

Physiologic adaptations in pregnancy prepare the patient for blood loss during the childbirth process. In addition to increased blood volume, serum clotting factors increase in pregnancy, including fibrinogen levels, von Willebrand factor, and levels of factors VII, VIII, IX, and X [25, 44]. Both inherited and acquired coagulation defects will predispose the patient to PPH.

Patients with inherited bleeding disorders require special care to prevent PPH [45]. Von Willebrand disease (vWD), the most common hereditary bleeding disorder, is present in approximately 1% of the population and may be mild or severe. Women with vWD may report a history of excessive menstrual bleeding [46]. Patients who are hemophilia carriers will have variable deficiencies in clotting factors; patients with the lowest concentrations of factor levels in the third trimester have higher incidence of PPH. Patients with known bleeding disorders are recommended to receive factor treatment prior to delivery to prevent PPH [45, 47]. In cases of PPH in patients with hereditary bleeding disorders, management involves replacement of deficient clotting factors [47].

Acquired bleeding disorders in the postpartum period include disseminated intravascular coagulation (DIC), quantitative platelet disorders including immune thrombocytopenic purpura (ITP), thrombotic thrombocytopenic purpura (TTP), and the HELLP syndrome of hemolysis, elevated liver enzymes, and low platelets [48].

DIC is a major concern in postpartum hemorrhage. DIC is a life-threatening consumptive coagulopathy that leads to microvascular thrombosis and may lead to organ failure. Exsanguinating PPH in the context of DIC is a complex syndrome involving consumption of coagulation factors and inability to stop bleeding after placental separation. Amniotic fluid contains procoagulants including a direct factor X activator as well as complement. An excess of tissue factor (TF) is released during detachment of the placenta from the uterine wall after delivery [49]. Placental tissue and syncytiotrophoblasts express higher levels of TF than other endothelial cells, and levels of TF are increased during the third trimester in a physiologic effort to prevent fibrinolysis. If TF is released into maternal circulation, as with placental abruption, amniotic fluid embolism, and placenta accreta, systemic activation rather than local activation of coagulation is initiated, leading to potentially widespread coagulation and depletion of platelets and fibrinogen [49]. Activation of the fibrinolytic system is followed by activation of the coagulation cascade [50]. Sepsis and infection can also lead to DIC through cytokine release [51].

Although characteristic laboratory features often define DIC, it is largely a clinical diagnosis. Identification of coagulopathy with labs including PT, PTT, fibrinogen, fibrin split products, D-dimer, and platelet levels may not be diagnostic in the patient in the immediate postpartum period. Typically, low fibrinogen levels are diagnostic of DIC for nonpregnant patients. However, fibrinogen is an acute-phase reactant and is unlikely to be low, even in pregnant or postpartum women with DIC, unless massive postpartum hemorrhage has occurred. It is important to trend fibrinogen levels in this setting, paying close attention to downward trends. D-dimer levels, which are normally elevated during pregnancy, are likely of little clinical value in bleeding pregnant or postpartum patients [49].

Emergency Department Management of Postpartum Hemorrhage

First-Line Treatments

Nearly all patients presenting to the ED with PPH will require simultaneous diagnostic evaluation and stabilization measures. Involvement of consultants from obstetrics and interventional radiology should be requested early in the course of care of the patient with PPH. The initial history and physical exam may provide insight into causes based on complications during pregnancy, history of bleeding, and cesarean versus vaginal delivery. Physical exam may reveal a boggy/atonic uterus or obvious traumatic laceration. Bimanual uterine compression during the initial examination may be therapeutic for controlling PPH. Initial laboratory tests include complete blood count, coagulation factors, and type and screen. Ultrasonography may reveal evidence for retained products of conception. If uterine inversion is detected, management involves placing the fundus back into the correct position. Gentle pressure on the uterine fundus with the palm of the hand as if holding a tennis ball will help correct positioning, but may require uterine relaxants such as magnesium and nitroglycerin to allow repositioning to occur [33, 52]. Pain should also be addressed. When PPH is severe, as indicated by observed volume of blood loss, an elevated shock index, or other markers such as elevated serum lactate, blood transfusion should be considered prior to a measurable fall in the patient's hemoglobin and hematocrit [19]. Emergency transfusion of uncrossmatched O negative blood or type-specific blood should be initiated as soon as severe PPH and hypovolemic shock are recognized [53].

If the uterus is palpably firm, or manual compression is not slowing bleeding, careful inspection of vaginal walls, cervix, and perineum should be completed for evaluation of tears or lacerations.

Pharmacologic Therapies

Several pharmaceuticals have the ability to stimulate the smooth muscle of the uterus. A familiarity with these agents, which are seldom used in the ED, can facilitate patient care during urgent situations involving PPH.

Oxytocin. Oxytocin, a synthetic formulation of the nonpeptide pituitary hormone, has stimulant effects on the smooth muscle of the uterus. Oxytocin stimulates uterine contractions by increasing intracellular calcium [54]. Oxytocin may be given prophylactically at the third stage of labor, and this has been shown to reduce PPH [55]. The initial dose is 10–40 units in 1000 ml crystalloid solution given as a continuous IV infusion [7] or up to 10 units intramuscular (IM). Rapid, undiluted IV administration should be avoided as this can cause hypotension. Oxytocin is the drug of choice for prophylaxis and treatment of PPH [56].

Methylergonovine. Midwives have used ergot alkaloids for centuries before being acknowledged by the medical profession in the mid-1800s. Ergot alkaloids directly stimulate uterine contraction. Methylergonovine is a semisynthetic ergot alkaloid that acts directly on the smooth muscle of the uterus and increases uterine contractions. The dose is 0.2 mg intramuscularly (IM) every 2–4 h [7], and onset of action is within minutes. Side effects include nausea and vomiting [55]. Methylergonovine should be avoided in women with a history of preeclampsia or coronary artery disease, as it can cause hypertension and vasospasm.

Prostaglandin analogs. Misoprostol is a prostaglandin E1 analog that induces contraction of the smooth muscle fibers of the myometrium. It can aid in contraction of the uterus to slow bleeding due to uterine atony [57]. It is used adjunctively in the management of retained placenta, but with inconclusive evidence as to its benefit over manual removal [30]. Misoprostol may be administered orally, buccally, sublingually, vaginally, or rectally with onset of action between 8 and 11 min when given via the oral or buccal route [58–60]. The recommended dose is 800–1000 mcg rectally [7]. When administered for postpartum hemorrhage, higher incidences of pyrexia have been described [61].

In cases of severe PPH, oxytocin, methylergonovine, and misoprostol may all be administered. Efficacies of methylergonovine and misoprostol each as single agents have not been found to be as efficacious as oxytocin alone [55, 62]. Misoprostol in conjunction with oxytocin to reduce PPH is associated with increased side effects of shivering and fever as compared to single therapy [62].

Desmopressin (DDAVP) is indicated in the management of PPH in patients with vWD and hemophilia carrier states; factor supplementation is indicated in patients with known deficiencies [47]. Factor VIIa administration has utility in patients with PPH complicated by coagulopathy, and antifibrinolytic therapy is an additional option for the prevention and control of PPH in patients with bleeding disorders [47, 63, 64]. The World Maternal Antifibrinolytic Trial (WOMAN Trial) of the use of tranexamic acid (TXA) has shown potential benefit for prevention of PPH in low-risk patients, but mixed reviews challenge its efficacy in the adjunctive treatment of active PPH [6, 64–66].

Second-Line Treatments: Mechanical and Surgical Interventions for PPH

Mechanical tamponade of uncontrolled uterine hemorrhage is necessary when bimanual massage, uterotonic drugs, and vaginal and uterine cavity examination fail to control PPH [67, 68]. Balloon tamponade, with digital insertion through the cervical os, is preferable to gauze packing [68]. Essentially any balloon device can be used to tamponade the bleeding. Bakri balloons, Sengstaken-Blakemore tubes, and Foley and condom catheters have demonstrated successful tamponade. Bakri balloons (Fig. 8.3) have been designed specifically for postpartum hemorrhage and allow for drainage of blood through side ports so active blood loss after insertion can be continuously assessed. The balloon should be filled with warm sterile water or saline. A vaginal pack is then placed to prevent balloon expulsion, and the balloon should remain for 24–48 h with simultaneous administration of uterotonics [68].

If Bakri balloons are not available, Foley or condom catheters or Blakemore tubes can be placed into the uterus and inflated to tamponade bleeding, typically with sterile saline to the maximum volume of the tube or when the uterine fundus is palpably firm. The proximal end of a urinary catheter must be occluded, typically with a silk tie, prior to insertion into the uterus and balloon inflation. The esophageal balloon of the Sengstaken-Blakemore tube has been shown to conform well to the shape of the uterus when compared to Foley catheters [69].

If balloon tamponade does not control PPH, invasive procedures must be considered. Uterine artery embolization is a therapeutic option for severe PPH refractory to conservative treatment measures [67, 70]. Uterine necrosis is a rare but serious complication [71]. Open vascular ligation and open compressive sutures (the

Fig. 8.3 Bakri balloon
tamponade device

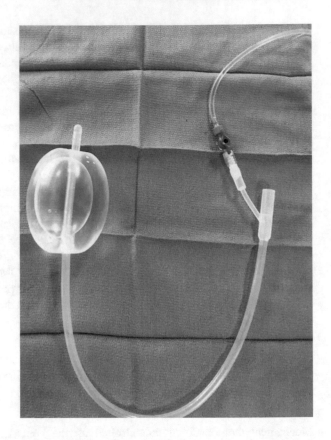

B-Lynch procedure) are emergency measures that may be required if interventional radiology is not available or medical therapy fails to control PPH [68]. Emergent hysterectomy is a procedure of last resort; it carries a high morbidity including DIC and ureter and bladder injury [72].

Emergency Department Disposition

The disposition of the patient from the ED after stabilization measures for PPH will be dependent on the resources available at the treating hospital and the hemodynamic stability of the patient. The majority of patients will require admission to an obstetrics unit. Stable patients with normal vital signs and complete resolution of bleeding can be observed for 8–12 h, monitoring hemoglobin and indices of coagulation. Patients with uncontrolled bleeding will require obstetric consultation and admission. Patients with hemodynamic instability or suspected DIC will require higher levels of care and intensive care monitoring. Hospitals without available obstetrics, general surgery, or interventional radiology on site will require transfer to a higher level of care, coordinating stabilization measures with the receiving hospital's specialty caregivers.

Summary

Postpartum hemorrhage can lead to severe blood loss and requires a unique set of emergency interventions to effectively treat the patient. Primary PPH occurs in the first 24 h after delivery, and secondary PPH occurs from 24 h up to 6–12 weeks postpartum. The most commonly identified etiologies of primary and secondary PPH include uterine atony and retained POC. Bimanual compression of the uterus is a first-line intervention and can be both diagnostic and therapeutic. Early recognition of maternal shock, early blood transfusion, and screening for coagulopathies can be life-saving. Uterotonic agents have utility in stimulating uterine contraction and reducing blood loss. Balloon tamponade is a bedside maneuver that may effectively control bleeding when conservative measures fail. More invasive measures such as uterine artery embolization and emergency hysterectomy may be required when first-line treatment measures fail to control PPH but carry significant risks of complications.

Key Points

- Postpartum hemorrhage can occur up to 6 weeks after delivery.
- Primary PPH is most commonly due to uterine atony, and secondary PPH is most often multifactorial, including atonic uterus, retained POC, and endometritis.
- Early signs of hemorrhagic shock, including a shock index greater than 0.9–1.1, should lead to consideration for blood transfusion, even before severe anemia is detected.
- Coagulopathies must be considered, and DIC may not initially present with lab abnormalities.
- Manual uterine compression and uterotonic drugs are first-line therapies, and endocavity balloon tamponade is a bedside procedure that may aid in control of hemorrhage.
- If medical therapies fail, uterine artery embolization or emergency hysterectomy may be necessary.
- Early involvement of obstetricians is crucial to patient survival.

References

1. Goffman D, Nathan L, Chazotte C. Obstetric hemorrhage: a global review. Semin Perinatol. 2016;40(2):96–8.
2. Bonnet MP, Benhamou D, Deneux-Tharaux C, Schmitz T. What is the true incidence of postpartum hemorrhage? Anesth Analg. 2015;121(5):1397.
3. Ekin A, Gezer C, Solmaz U, et al. Predictors of severity in primary postpartum hemorrhage. Arch Gynecol Obstet. 2015;292(6):1247–54.
4. Creanga A, Berg C, Syverson C. Pregnancy-related mortality in the United States 2006-2010. Obstet Gynecol. 2015;125(1):5–12.
5. Abdul-Kadir R, McLintock C, Ducloy A, et al. Evaluation and management of postpartum hemorrhage: consensus from an international expert panel. Transfusion. 2014;54(7):1756–68.

6. Shakur H, Elbourne D, Gulmezoglu M, et al. The WOMAN Trial (World Maternal Antifibrinolytic Trial): tranexamic acid for the treatment of postpartum haemorrhage: an international randomized, double blind placebo controlled trial. Trials. 2010;11:40.
7. American College of Obstetricians and Gynecologists. ACOG Practice Bulletin: clinical management guidelines for obstetrician-gynecologists number 76, October 2006: postpartum hemorrhage. Obstet Gynecol. 2006;108(4):1039–47.
8. Golmakani N, Khaleghinezhad K, Dadgar S, et al. Comparing the estimation of postpartum hemorrhage using the weighing method and National Guideline with the postpartum hemorrhage estimation by midwives. Iran J Nurs Midwifery Res. 2015;20(4):471–5.
9. Saad A, Costantine MM. Obstetric hemorrhage: recent advances. Clin Obstet Gynecol. 2014;57(4):791–6.
10. ACOG. http://www.acog.org/. Accessed 30 June 2016.
11. Ajenifuja KO, Adepiti CA, Ogunniyi SO. Postpartum hemorrhage in a teaching hospital in Nigeria: a 5-year experience. Afr Health Sci. 2010;10(1):71–4.
12. Kominiarek M, Kilpatrick S. Postpartum hemorrhage: a recurring pregnancy complication. Semin Perinatol. 2007;31:159–66.
13. Rath WH. Postpartum hemorrhage – update on problems of definitions and diagnosis. Acta Obstet Gynecol Scand. 2011;90(5):421–8.
14. Stafford I, Dildy GA, Clark SL, Belfort MA. Visually estimated and calculated blood loss in vaginal and cesarean delivery. Am J Obstet Gynecol. 2008;199:519.e1–7.
15. Warrilow G, Kirkham C, Ismail K, et al. Quantification of menstrual blood loss. Obstet Gynecol. 2004;6:88–92.
16. Patel A, Goudar SS, Geller SE, et al. drape estimation vs visual assessment for estimating postpartum hemorrhage. Int J Gynaecol Obstet. 2006;93(3):220–4.
17. Kramer MS, Berg C, Abenhaim H, et al. Incidence, risk factors and temporal trends in severe postpartum hemorrhage. Am J Obstet Gynecol. 2013;209:449.e1–7.
18. El Ayadi A, Nathan H, Seed P, et al. Vital sign prediction of adverse maternal outcomes in women with hypovolemic shock: the role of shock index. PLoS One. 2016;11(2):e0148. 729
19. Clark S. Obstetric hemorrhage. Semin Perinatol. 2016;40:109–11.
20. Le Bas A, Chandraharan E, Addei A, Arulkumaran S. Use of the "obstetric shock index" as an adjunct in identifying significant blood loss in patients with massive postpartum hemorrhage. Int J Gynaecol Obstet. 2014;124(3):253–5.
21. Sohn CH, Kim WY, Kim SR, et al. An increase in initial shock index is associated with the requirement for massive transfusion in emergency department patients with primary postpartum hemorrhage. Shock. 2013;40(2):101–5.
22. Goodwin S, Spies J. Uterine fibroid embolization. N Engl J Med. 2009;161:690–7.
23. Frolova A, Stout M, Tuuli M, et al. Duration of the third stage of labor and risk of postpartum hemorrhage. Obstet Gynecol. 2016;127:951–6.
24. Wetta L, Szychowski J, Seals S, et al. Risk factors for uterine atony/postpartum hemorrhage requiring treatment after vaginal delivery. Am J Obstet Gynecol. 2013;209:51.e1–6.
25. Friedman A. Obstetric hemorrhage. J Cardiothorac Vasc Anesth. 2013;27(245):s44–8.
26. Breathnach F, Geary M. Uterine Atony: definition, prevention, nonsurgical management, and uterine tamponade. Semin Perinatol. 2009;33(2):82–7.
27. Chan L, Lo T, Lau W, et al. Use of second-line therapies for management of massive primary postpartum hemorrhage. Int J Gynaecol Obstet. 2013;122:238–43.
28. Blomberg M. Maternal obesity and risk of postpartum hemorrhage. Obstet Gynecol. 2011;118(3):561–8.
29. Andreatta P, Perosky J, Johnson TR. Two-provider technique for bimanual uterine compression to control postpartum hemorrhage. J Midwifery Womens Health. 2012;57(4):371–5.
30. Grillo-Ardila CF, Ruiz-Parra AI, Gaitán HG, Rodriguez-Malagon N. Prostaglandins for management of retained placenta. Cochrane Database Syst Rev. 2014;(5). Art. No.: CD010312.
31. Van Beekhuizen H, Tarimo V, Pembe AB, et al. A randomized controlled trial on the value of misoprostol for the treatment of retained placenta in a low-resource setting. Int J Gynecol Obstet. 2013;3(122):234–7.

32. Oyelese Y, Ananth C. Postpartum hemorrhage: epidemiology, risk factors and causes. Clin Obstet Gynecol. 2010;53(1):147–56.
33. Leal R, Mano Luz R, Pinto de Almeida J, et al. Total and acute uterine inversion after delivery: a case report. J Med Case Reports. 2014;8:347.
34. Bhalla R, Wuntakal R, Odejinmi F, Khan R. Acute inversion of the uterus. Obstet Gynecol. 2009;11:13–8.
35. Kawano H, Hasegawa J, Nakamura M, et al. Upside-down and inside-out signs in uterine inversion. J Clin Med Res. 2016;8(7):548–9.
36. Dossou M, Debost-Legrand A, Dechelotte P, et al. Severe secondary postpartum hemorrhage: a historical cohort. Birth. 2015;42(2):149–55.
37. Sellmyer M, Desser T, Maturen K. Physiologic, histologic and imaging features of retained products of conception. Radiographics. 2013;33:781–96.
38. Zubor P, Kajo K, Dokus K, et al. Recurrent secondary postpartum hemorrhages due to placental site vessel subinvolution and local uterine tissue coagulopathy. BMC Pregnancy Childbirth. 2014;14:80. http://www.biomedcentral.com/1471-2392/14/80
39. Petrovitch I, Jeffery R, Heerema-McKenney A. Subinvolution of the placental site. J Ultrasound Med. 2009;28(8):1115–9.
40. Robye C, Petersen IS, Nilas L. Postpartum Clostridium sordellii infection associated with fatal toxic shock syndrome. Acta Obstet Gynecol Scand. 2000;79(12):1134–5.
41. Mackeen AD, Packard RE, Ota E, Speer L. Antibiotic regimens for postpartum endometritis. Cochrane Database Syst Rev. 2015;2:CD001067.
42. Chitra TV, Panicker S. Pseudoaneurysm of uterine artery: a rare cause of secondary postpartum hemorrhage. J Obstet Gynaecol India. 2011;61(6):641–4.
43. Yeniel AO, Ergenoglu AM, Eminov E, et al. Massive secondary postpartum hemorrhage with uterine artery pseudoaneurysm after cesarean section. Case Rep Obstet Gynecol. 2013; ID285846.
44. Girard T, Mortl M, Schlembach D. New approaches to obstetric hemorrhage: the postpartum hemorrhage consensus algorithm. Curr Opin Anesthesiol. 2014;27(3):267–74.
45. Stoof SC, van Steenbergen HW, Zwagemaker A, et al. Primary postpartum hemorrhage in women with von Willebrand disease or carriership of haemophilia despite specialized care: a retrospective survey. Hemophilia. 2015;21(4):505–12.
46. Stefanska E, Vertun-Baranowska B, Windyga J, Lopaciuk S. Von Willebrand disease in women with menorrhagia. Ginekol Pol. 2004;75(1):47–52.
47. Kouides P. An update on the management of bleeding disorders during pregnancy. Curr Opin Hematol. 2015;22(5):397–405.
48. James AH, Cooper DL, Paidas MJ. Hemostatic assessment, treatment strategies and hematology consultation in massive postpartum hemorrhage: results of a quantitative survey of obstetrician-gynecologists. Int J Womens Health. 2015;4(7):873–81.
49. Erez O, Mastrolia SA, Thachil J. Disseminated intravascular coagulation in pregnancy: insights in pathophysiology, diagnosis and management. Am J Obstet Gynecol. 2015;213(4):452–63.
50. Montagnana M, Franchi M, Danese E, et al. Disseminated intravascular coagulation in obstetric and gynecologic disorders. Semin Thromb Hemost. 2010;36(4):404–18.
51. Van der Poll T, de Jonge E, Levi M. Regulatory role of cytokines in disseminated intravascular coagulation. Semin Thromb Hemost. 2001;27(6):639–51.
52. Bullarbo M, Bokström H, Lilja H, et al. Nitroglycerin for management of retained placenta: a multicenter study. Obstet Gynecol Int. 2012. Article ID 321207, 6 ps, doi: 10.1155/2012/321207.
53. Fleischer A, Meirowitz N. Care bundles for management of obstetrical hemorrhage. Semin Perinatol. 2016;40(2):99–108.
54. Arrowsmith S, Wray S. Oxytocin: its mechanism of action and receptor signaling in the myometrium. J Neuroendocrinol. 2014;26(6):356–69.
55. Westhoff G, Cotter AM, Tolosa JE. Prophylactic oxytocin for the third stage of labour to prevent postpartum haemorrhage. Cochrane Database Syst Rev. 2013;(10). Art. No.: CD001808. doi: 10.1002/14651858.CD001808.pub2.

56. Gizzo S, Patrelli TS, Gangi SD, et al. Which uterotonic is better to prevent the postpartum hemorrhage? Latest in terms of clinical efficacy, side effects, and contraindications. Reprod Sci. 2013;20(9):1011–9.
57. Marret H, Simon E, Beucher G, et al. Overview and expert assessment of off-label use of misoprostol in obstetrics and gynaecology. Eur J Obstet Gyn Reprod Biol. 2015;187:80–4.
58. Tang OS, Gemzell-Danielsson K, Ho PC. Misoprostol: pharmacokinetic profiles, effects on the uterus and side effects. Int J Gynecol Obstet. 2007;99(Suppl 2):S160–7.
59. Chaudhuri P, Mandi S, Mazumdar A. Rectally administrated misoprostol as an alternative to intravenous oxytocin infusion for preventing post-partum hemorrhage after cesarean delivery. J Obstet Gynaecol Res. 2014;40(9):2023–30.
60. Sheldon WR, Blum J, Durocher J, Winikoff B. Misoprostol for the prevention and treatment of postpartum hemorrhage. Expert Opin Investig Drugs. 2012;21(2):235–50.
61. Weeks A, Nielson J. Rethinking our approach to postpartum haemorrhage and uterotonics. BMJ. 2015;351:1–5.
62. Tunçalp Ö, Souza J, Gulmezoglu M. New WHO recommendations on prevention and treatment of postpartum hemorrhage. Int J Gyn Ogstet. 2013;123:254–46.
63. Baudo F, Caimi TM, Mostarda G, et al. Critical bleeding in pregnancy: a novel therapeutic approach to bleeding. Minerva Anestesiol. 2006;72(6):389–93.
64. Ekelund K, Hanke G, Stensballe J, et al. Hemostatic resuscitation in postpartum hemorrhage: a supplement to surgery. Acta Obstet Gynecol Scand. 2015;94(7):680–92.
65. Novikova N, Hofmeyr G, Cluver C. Tranexamic acid for preventing bleeding after delivery. Cochrane Database Syst Rev. 2015;(6). Art. No.: CD007872. Accessed 12 July 2016.
66. Sujata N, Tobin R, Kaur R, et al. Randomized controlled trial of tranexamic acid among parturients at increased risk for postpartum hemorrhage undergoing cesarean delivery. Int J Gynaecol Obstet. 2016;133(3):312–5.
67. Winograd RH. Uterine artery embolization for postpartum hemorrhage. Best Pract Res Clin Obstet Gynaecol. 2008;22(6):1119–32.
68. Lombaard H, Pattinson R. Common errors and remedies in managing postpartum haemorrhage. Best Pract Res Clin Obstet Gynaecol. 2009;23:317–26.
69. Georgiou C. Balloon tamponade in the management of postpartum haemorrhage: a review. BJOG. 2009;116:748–57.
70. Vegas G, Illescas T, Munoz M, Perez-Pinar A. Selective pelvic arterial embolization in the management of obstetric hemorrhage. Eur J Obstet Gynecol Reprod Biol. 2006;127(1):68–72.
71. Poujade O, Ceccaldi PF, Davitian C, et al. Uterine necrosis following pelvic arterial embolization for postpartum hemorrhage. Eur J Obstet Gynecol Reprod Biol. 2013;170(2):309–14.
72. Yamani Zamzami TY. Indication of emergency peripartum hysterectomy: review of 17 cases. Arch Gynecol Obstet. 2003;268(3):131–5.

Chapter 9
Cardiovascular Emergencies of Pregnancy

Lisel Curtis and Nick Tsipis

Introduction

Cardiovascular emergencies in pregnancy, while rare, can be catastrophic for mother and fetus. The unique physiologic changes of pregnancy are demanding on the cardiovascular system and place pregnant patients at increased risk for potentially lethal complications including venous thromboembolism, aortic dissection, and peripartum cardiomyopathy (PPCM). Diagnosis of these three conditions is difficult as signs and symptoms overlap with each other and can also be experienced in normal pregnancies. Evaluation of the pregnant patient with a cardiovascular emergency comes with unique challenges; ionizing radiation exposure to mother and fetus must be considered when selecting an imaging modality, and certain drugs are contraindicated in pregnancy. Managing a critically ill pregnant patient is stressful for the entire emergency department team as two lives are at stake. Providers must remember that the best chance of fetal survival is maternal survival. A coordinated response by a team that includes obstetricians, surgeons, anesthesiologists, and neonatologists will optimize outcomes for both mother and fetus. It is incumbent on the emergency physician to make an accurate and timely diagnosis, lead resuscitative efforts, and coordinate the interdisciplinary care team.

L. Curtis, M.D. (✉)
Department of Emergency Medicine, MedStar Georgetown University Hospital,
3800 Reservoir Road, NW, Washington, DC 20007, USA
e-mail: lieslcurtis@gmail.com

N. Tsipis, M.D.
Department of Emergency Medicine, MedStar Georgetown University Hospital and MedStar Washington Hospital Center, 3800 Reservoir Road, NW, Washington, DC 20007, USA
e-mail: nick.tsipis@gmail.com

© Springer International Publishing AG 2017
J. Borhart (ed.), *Emergency Department Management of Obstetric Complications*,
DOI 10.1007/978-3-319-54410-6_9

Venous Thromboembolism (VTE) in Pregnancy

Venous thromboembolism (VTE) is a disease that includes both deep venous thrombosis (DVT) and pulmonary embolism (PE). Hormonal and physiologic changes that occur in the body during pregnancy including hypercoagulability, venous stasis, decreased venous outflow, mechanical compression of the inferior vena cava (IVC) and pelvic veins by the gravid uterus, and decreased mobility place the pregnant patient at higher risk for VTE [1]. There is up to a tenfold increase risk of a thromboembolic event in pregnancy than in the nonpregnant state, and over one half occur in the third trimester [2]. An increased rate of thrombosis exists until 12 weeks postpartum, but is greatest during the first 3–6 weeks postpartum [3]. When considering risk factors for a thromboembolic event in pregnancy, the most important risk factors are a prior history of DVT/PE and the pre-existing history of a thrombophilia [4, 5]. Thromboembolic events are a leading cause of mortality in pregnancy; PE represented 9.8% of pregnancy-related deaths in 2011 [6].

Deep Vein Thrombosis

DVTs in pregnancy tend to be proximal and large and in the left lower extremity. The left-sided location is thought to be due to the compression of the left common iliac vein by the right common iliac artery and the gravid uterus [4]. Compression ultrasonography is still the first approach in the evaluation of DVT in pregnancy. However, a negative ultrasound doesn't completely exclude a DVT as pelvic DVTs are more common in pregnancy and are often missed on ultrasound. If iliac vein thrombosis is suspected and the ultrasound is negative, the American College of Obstetricians and Gynecologists (ACOG) recommends proceeding to a non-contrast MRI [1]. Serial ultrasounds can be performed in patients with a negative ultrasound, but in whom the clinician has a high clinical concern of DVT. Additionally, ultrasound can be used as a first step even if PE is the primary concern. If a DVT is found, treatment can begin without the need for computed tomography pulmonary angiography (CTPA) or ventilation/perfusion (V/Q) scan (Fig. 9.1).

Pulmonary Embolism

The diagnosis of PE is difficult in the pregnant patient as the clinical signs and symptoms of PE (dyspnea, tachycardia, lower extremity edema) occur in normal pregnancy. Clinical decision rules have barely been studied in pregnant patients, and none have been validated in the pregnant population. Standard diagnostic tools such as D-dimer lose accuracy as levels increase physiologically during normal pregnancy. As such, physicians tend to test for PE at lower thresholds in pregnant patients and rely heavily on diagnostic imaging studies. Indeed, the incidence of PE is 5% or less in most studies of pregnant patients with suspected PE, compared to 20–25% in nonpregnant patients [7]. Several diagnostic algorithms have been proposed, but the optimal strategy to diagnose PE in pregnancy remains under debate.

Fig. 9.1 Ultrasound image of decreased blood flow through right femoral vein DVT in transverse view. Reprinted with permission of the MedStar Georgetown University Hospital & MedStar Washington Hospital Center Emergency Ultrasound Group

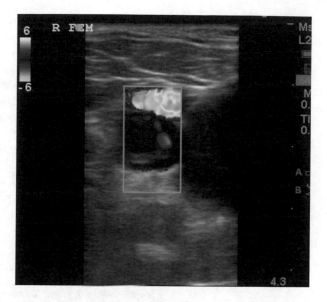

The D-dimer represents a breakdown product of cross-linked fibrin and is a useful screening tool for DVT/PE in the nonpregnant population. In pregnancy, however, the D-dimer level increases steadily with each trimester, making the test less useful to rule out VTE. Multiple studies have evaluated trimester-adjusted thresholds for normal D-dimer levels in pregnancy, but results are inconsistent [8–12]. Even if "normal range" pregnancy values are firmly established, the threshold to safely exclude VTE would need to be identified. Some authors and guidelines state that a negative D-dimer is still reliably negative in a pregnant patient with low pretest probability [13, 14]. Other guidelines are contradictory and conclude that the D-dimer cannot currently be used to exclude suspected PE in pregnancy [15].

The diagnostic work-up of patients with suspected PE often begins assessment of pretest probability using a validated clinical decision rule. The modified Wells score (MWS) is a validated clinical tool (in nonpregnant patients) used to risk stratify patients in whom there is clinical concern for PE (Table 9.1). It is often used in conjunction with a D-dimer to guide the work-up.

Several studies have evaluated the MWS in pregnancy. A retrospective review by O'Connor et al. [17] applied the MWS to 81 pregnant and 22 postpartum patients referred for CTPA over a 5-year period. The authors found that an MWS of 6 or greater was 100% sensitive and 90% specific with a positive predictive value of 36% for PE on CTPA. This study is small and retrospective and lacked follow-up data, but shows a promising application of the MWS in pregnant patients.

A second study by Parilla et al. [12] evaluated trimester-specific D-dimer levels combined with the MWS as useful risk stratification tools in pregnant women in a prospective and retrospective cohort study. While the number of patients included in the study was low, the results were promising. Using both trimester-specific D-dimers and an MWS was 100% sensitive and 81.4% specific in detecting PE if either of the results were abnormal. In this study, all of the patients with PE would have received a CTPA, and the total number of CTPAs performed would have been decreased by 52.5%.

Currently, imaging tests are the mainstay of diagnostic management of suspected PE in pregnancy. When choosing an imaging modality, risks to the fetus and mother must be considered. The two most commonly used studies for suspected PE are CTPA and V/Q scan. VQ scan confers a higher dose of radiation to the fetus, while CTPA delivers more radiation to the mother, particularly to breast tissue. Breast tissue of pregnant women has a high rate of cell turnover and thus more susceptible to ionizing radiation. However, CTPA can identify alternate pathology. Both forms of imaging confer radiation doses much lower than the exposure associated with fetal harm (Table 9.2).

Multiple diagnostic algorithms for suspected PE in pregnancy have been proposed. The American Thoracic Society and the Society of Thoracic Radiology published one such clinical practice guideline in 2011 [15]. A multidisciplinary panel including members of ACOG was convened to develop evidence-based recommen-

Table 9.1 Modified Wells score[a]—prediction rule for diagnosing PE

Clinical symptoms of DVT	3
Other diagnosis less likely than PE	3
Pulse >100	1.5
Immobilization ≥3 days or surgery in previous 4 weeks	1.5
Previous PE or DVT	1.5
Hemoptysis	1
Malignancy	1
Low probability	0–1
Intermediate probability	2–6
High probability	>6

[a]Modified from Chagnon I, et al. Comparison of Two Clinical Prediction Rules and Implicit Assessment among Patients with Suspected Pulmonary Embolism. Am J Med. 2002 [16]

Table 9.2 VQ scan vs. CTPA for evaluation of pulmonary embolism

	VQ scan	CTPA
Fetal radiation exposure[a]	0.37 mGy dose Radiation exposure greater to fetus	0.01–0.66 mGy Radiation exposure greater to mother, especially maternal breast tissue
Iodinated contrast exposure	N/A	Contrast exposure with possible induction of neonatal hypothyroidism; FDA classifies iodinated contrast as "B" level recommendation for safety
Diagnostic value	Rate of nondiagnostic study is between 7 and 21%	Can identify pathology other than PE

[a]Fetal exposure varies with gestational age, maternal body habitus. Data from: Dubbs SB, Tewelde SZ. Cardiovascular catastrophes in the obstetric population. Emerg Med Clin North Am. 2015;33:483–500. Winer-Muram HT, et al. Pulmonary embolism in pregnant patients: fetal radiation dose with helical CT. Radiology 2002;224:487–92. American College of Obstetricians and Gynecologists' Committee on Obstetric Practice. Committee Opinion No. 656: Guidelines for Diagnostic Imaging During Pregnancy and Lactation. *Obstet Gynecol.* 2016. *CTPA* computed tomographic pulmonary angiogram, *V/Q* ventilation perfusion

dations. Overall, the panel found that there was "limited amount of direct evidence pertaining to diagnostic test accuracy and patient-important outcomes in the pregnant population." Nonetheless, recommendations were made and are summarized in Fig. 9.2. If the patient has leg symptoms (swelling, calf pain, or asymmetry), bilateral lower extremity ultrasounds to evaluate for DVT should be the starting point. If a DVT is found, begin treatment without further work-up. If there are no leg symptoms, the first step in the evaluation of a PE should be a chest X-ray (CXR) as it may show other etiologies that explain the patient's symptoms (e.g., pneumonia, pulmonary edema). In the pregnant patient with a normal CXR and no history of pulmonary disease (such as asthma), V/Q scan is recommended. If the patient has an abnormal CXR or a history of pulmonary disease, CTPA is recommended.

Other algorithms have been proposed and clinical practice varies widely. Several authors recommend obtaining bilateral lower extremity ultrasounds as a first step when either DVT or PE is suspected [18, 19]. If chest imaging is necessary, the authors believe both CTPA and V/Q scans are equally justifiable for the pregnant patient. The authors prefer CTPA as it may identify alternate pathology. Additionally, there is a risk that the V/Q scan may be indeterminate, requiring that a CTPA be performed as well (Fig. 9.3).

Once the diagnosis of PE/DVT is made in a pregnant patient, treatment with either low molecular weight heparin (LMWH) or unfractionated heparin (UFH) is

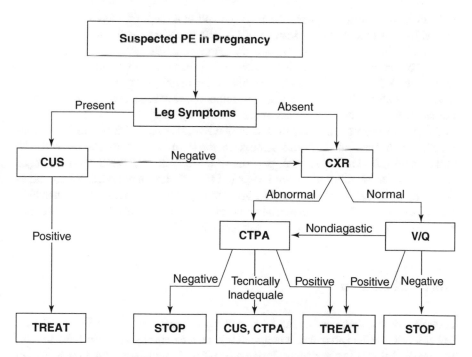

Fig. 9.2 Diagnostic algorithm for suspected PE in pregnancy. (Reprinted with permission of the American Thoracic Society. Copyright © 2016 American Thoracic Society. Leung AN, et al. [15]. The *American Journal of Respiratory and Critical Care Medicine* is an official journal of the American Thoracic Society. *CUS* compression ultrasonography, *CXR* chest X-ray, *CTPA* computed tomographic pulmonary angiogram, *V/Q* ventilation perfusion)

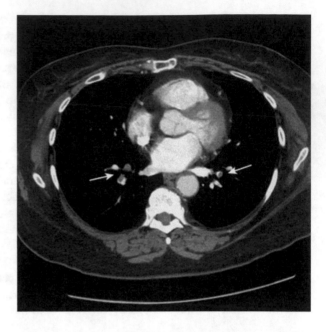

Fig. 9.3 CTPA revealing intraluminal filling defects (*arrows*) in the pulmonary vascular tree. From Sibai BM, eds. *Management of Acute Obstetric Emergencies*. Philadelphia: Saunders, 2011; With permission

indicated. Neither drug crosses the placenta and both are considered safe in pregnancy. UFH is recommended instead of LMWH in patients with GFR less than 30 mL/min or in situations where delivery, surgery, or thrombolysis is imminent. Thrombolytic therapy should be considered for pregnant women with life- or limbthreatening VTE [20]. Warfarin is contraindicated in pregnancy because it is associated with teratogenic fetal effects. To the authors' knowledge, there is no controlled human data regarding novel anticoagulants and pregnancy.

Disposition of pregnant patients with newly diagnosed VTE is similar to nonpregnant patients, but decisions should be made in close consultation with the patient's obstetrician. In general, patients who are clinically stable with no major risk factors for bleeding and easy access to medical care may be treated as outpatients. Hospitalization is indicated in patients who are hemodynamically unstable and have extensive VTE or maternal comorbidities that increase their risk of major bleeding or in patients that require treatment with UFH.

Aortic Dissection

A rare but devastating cardiovascular emergency of pregnancy is a major vessel arterial dissection. While an overall uncommon event, the majority of aortic dissections in women of childbearing age occur during pregnancy. Indeed, for women younger than 40, pregnancy is associated with a markedly increased risk of aortic dissection (odds ratio of 25) [21]. The role of the emergency physician includes early recognition, resuscitation, early activation of institutional massive transfusion protocols, immediate surgical and obstetrical consultation, and overall coordination of care.

The well-described physiologic and hemodynamic changes of pregnancy in concert with accompanying hormonal changes create significant new stresses on the circulatory systems. The gravid uterus compresses the abdominal aorta and iliac arteries, leading to increased vascular resistance at the point of compression and increased stress on the intimal layers of the more proximal aorta. It is suspected that these stresses, in combination with increased effective circulating volume, heart rate, cardiac output, and other hemodynamic changes of pregnancy, create new strains on the vasculature of even previously healthy pregnant patients. The role of elevated progesterone and, more importantly, estrogen augments these hemodynamic stresses. As early as the first trimester, maternal arterial vessels begin to demonstrate increased compliance [22]. Postmortem histopathologic examination from fatal aortic dissections in pregnant patients demonstrates severe degeneration of elastin fibers and other markers of "arterial degeneration" [23]. Patients with known connective tissue disorders or conditions (Ehlers-Danlos, Marfan's, and Turner's syndromes) are also at increased risk for acute aortic dissection.

A recent nationwide study from the Netherlands [24] examined vascular dissections causing death in 23 pregnant patients (incidence 0.74 per 100,000 live births). The authors observed the most frequent location of dissection to be the aorta, with coronary and splenic artery dissections less common. The clinical presentation for a thoracic aortic dissection was variable, but the majority of patients had classic complaints of severe, sharp chest pain described as "ripping" and/or "tearing" and radiating to the back, sometimes accompanied by nausea and vomiting. However, making the diagnosis is challenging. Undoubtedly, the clinical presentation of dissections often significantly overlaps with other cardiovascular emergencies in the pregnant patient such as PE, acute coronary disease, amniotic fluid embolism, or preeclampsia. As described previously in the VTE section, D-dimer is not a useful screening tool as levels rise steadily throughout normal pregnancy.

To definitively diagnose aortic dissection, imaging is required. Similar to nonpregnant patients, CT or transesophageal electrocardiography (TEE) may be used. TEE is ideal in pregnancy as it confers no ionizing radiation and can be performed in the ED, but is not always available. CT does confer ionizing radiation and requires intravenous contrast; however, these risks must be weighed against the risks of missing a potentially lethal vascular catastrophe. Importantly, a necessary diagnostic test should not be withheld from a pregnant patient out of concern for possible risk to the fetus. Bedside ultrasonography may also be useful. Findings such as intimal flaps within the abdominal aorta, grossly dilated vascular size, a false lumen, or hemopericardium warrant emergent angiography or other more immediate action depending on the patient's hemodynamic status (Fig. 9.4).

For thoracic aortic dissections, management depends on its location. Type A (proximal/ascending) dissections require emergent surgical intervention with fetal monitoring. If the fetus has reached viability (>23 weeks), delivery via caesarian should be considered prior to vascular surgical repair as cardiac surgery is associated with increased fetal loss. Medical management is preferred for uncomplicated type B dissections. Endovascular procedures are being used now in complicated type B dissections [25].

In the patient without aortic rupture but confirmed dissection, ED management includes lowering the heart rate then blood pressure while maintaining clinical indicators

Fig. 9.4 Transverse view of aortic dissection with flap and false lumen in a patient with Marfan's. Reprinted with permission of the MedStar Georgetown University Hospital & MedStar Washington Hospital Center Emergency Ultrasound Group

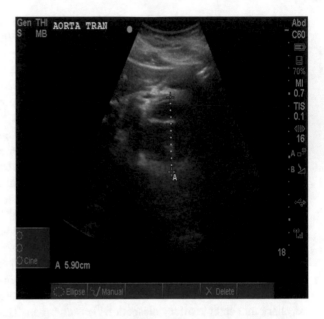

of adequate perfusion. Vasodilation without beta-blockade can cause reflex tachycardia, increase sheer stress on the damaged intima, and potentially paradoxically worsen extension of the false lumen. Labetalol, nitroprusside, nitroglycerin, and nicardipine all available as infusions are the agents of choice (Table 9.3). Higher doses than usual may be required due to the higher baseline sympathetic drive of pregnancy. All patients with acute aortic dissections required hospital admission, usually to an intensive care unit.

Peripartum Cardiomyopathy

The pregnant or postpartum patient presenting with progressive dyspnea and/or chest discomfort may be manifesting the development of peripartum cardiomyopathy (PPCM), also referred to as pregnancy-associated cardiomyopathy or pregnancy-associated heart failure. Though several working definitions of PPCM exist, one of the most inclusive was defined in 2010 by the European Society of Cardiology (ESC) as an "idiopathic cardiomyopathy presenting with heart failure secondary to left-ventricular (LV) systolic dysfunction towards the end of pregnancy or in the months following delivery, where no other cause of heart failure is found" [26]. The incidence of PPCM in the USA is relatively low (estimates range from 1:2500–4000 to 0.1%) but carries considerable morbidity and mortality, ranging from 5 to 32% [27]. Cardiology and obstetric consultation should be sought early in the ED course of a patient with PPCM.

Risk factors for the development of PPCM include those classically associated with the development of cardiovascular disease (hypertension, diabetes, tobacco use) as well as pregnancy-specific factors (e.g., advanced maternal age, multiparity, multiple pregnancies, use of tocolytics, nutritional status). The exact cause of PPCM is not clear. Proposed mechanisms of the pathophysiology of PPCM include viral

Table 9.3 Profiles of common cardiovascular medications available during pregnancy

Action	Medication	Considerations
Afterload reduction	Hydralazine	Safe and well studied in pregnancy. Often chosen first
	Nitrates (isosorbide mononitrate, nitroglycerin, nitroprusside)	Commonly used and considered safe, but pose a theoretic risk of cyanide toxicity (nitroprusside)
	Calcium channel blocker	Not first-line/preferred therapy, only nifedipine has been shown to be safe in pregnancy
	ACE inhibitors ARBs	*Contraindicated* in pregnancy, but first choice in postpartum patients
Preload reduction	Loop diuretics	Most likely necessary; can cause decreased placental blood flow
	Nitrates (isosorbide mononitrate, nitroglycerin, nitroprusside)	Commonly used and considered safe, but pose a theoretic risk of cyanide toxicity (nitroprusside)
	Spironolactone (aldosterone antagonist)	Avoid during pregnancy—believed to have androgenic effects in the first trimester
β-Blockers	Metoprolol, labetolol	Considered safe; some evidence of IUGR; β-1 selective preferred because β-2 receptor blockade can theoretically have an anti-tocolytic action
Anticoagulants	Coumadin	Contraindicated in pregnancy; potential for teratogenicity as well as pregnancy loss
	Low molecular weight heparin	Preferred anticoagulant in pregnant women with acute VTE
	Unfractionated heparin	Use if patient's GFR < 30 mL/min; use if anticipate thrombolysis, urgent surgery or delivery

Adapted from: Sommerkamp SK, Gibson A. Cardiovascular disasters in pregnancy. Emerg Med Clin North Am. 2012;30:952. Sahni G. Chest Pain Syndromes in Pregnancy. Cardiol Clin 30 (2012) 343–367
ACE angiotensin-converting enzyme, *ARB* angiotensin-receptor blockers, *VTE* venous thrombo-embolism, *GFR* glomerular filtration rate, *IUGR* intrauterine growth restriction

myocarditis, abnormal immune response to pregnancy, abnormal response to the hemodynamic stress of pregnancy, and possibly genetic factors [28].

The majority of patients develop symptoms in the first 4 months after delivery, with 75% of cases diagnosed in the first month postpartum [29]. Symptoms of PPCM are the same for typical heart failure, including pedal edema, dyspnea on exertion, orthopnea, paroxysmal nocturnal dyspnea, persistent cough, abdominal pain from hepatic congestion, dizziness, chest pain, and palpitations. PPCM can be difficult to diagnose because, like PE and dissection, many of the symptoms overlap with the normal physiologic changes of pregnancy. Normal pregnancy, with increased blood volume, increased metabolic demands, mild anemia, changes in vascular resistance associated with mild ventricular dilatation, and increased cardiac output, can mimic the early signs and symptoms of PPCM. Some patients may present with acutely decompensated heart failure, with New York Heart Association class III or IV symptoms (symptoms with minimal exertion or at rest) [30].

Evaluation of potential PPCM is multimodal in an attempt to delineate heart failure from PE, acute coronary syndrome, thoracic aortic dissection, or preeclampsia. Electrocardiography is often abnormal, with 66% of patients with PPCM showing left ventricular hypertrophy and nearly all demonstrating some degree of ST-T wave abnormality [31]. CXR can confirm pulmonary congestion or reveal another etiology of shortness of breath such as pneumonia or pleural effusions. Echocardiography is the most important study and should be performed in all patients suspected of having PPCM. The ejection fraction (EF) is nearly always reduced below 45%, though there may not be left ventricular dilation [26]. Laboratory tests such as brain natriuretic peptide (BNP) may be helpful in ruling in or out heart failure. Additional labs such as complete blood count, complete metabolic profile, and urinalysis may help distinguish PPCM from preeclampsia.

Management of heart failure in the pregnant patient depends on severity of the disease and is similar to the treatment of nonpregnant patients. An important exception is the choice of pharmacologic agents. While diuretics, beta-blockers, angiotensin-converting enzyme (ACE) inhibitors, angiotensin-receptor blockers (ARBs), hydralazine plus nitrates, and aldosterone antagonists have all demonstrated prolonged survival in nonpregnant patients, ACE inhibitors, ARBs, and aldosterone antagonists are associated with harmful fetal effects and are contraindicated in pregnant patients. Also, atenolol has been linked to fetal growth restriction [32]. In general, agents that preferentially act as beta-1 receptors vs. beta-2 are preferable so as to not inhibit beta-2-mediated uterine relaxation and peripheral vasodilation. Diuretics may be necessary, but should be used with caution in pregnant patients as maternal volume depletion can lead to uteroplacental hypoperfusion. Critically ill patients may require noninvasive ventilation support or intubation. Patients that experience refractory or a devastating initial presentation of heart failure during pregnancy with a suspected reversible cause can be candidates for specific advanced therapy, including an intra-aortic balloon pump (IABP) or extracorporeal membrane oxygenation (ECMO) to provide maximal circulatory support. Additionally, these patients can be candidates for mechanical support devices like left ventricular assist devices (LVADs) as either a bridge to cardiac transplant or permanent therapy. Bromocriptine, a dopamine 2 agonist that blocks the release of prolactin and aims to combat prolactin split product cardiotoxicity, has prevented onset of PPCM in several animal models and is being studied with ongoing prospective randomized control trials. A small "proof-of-concept" study adding bromocriptine to the standard heart failure therapy showed promising results of improved left ventricular ejection fraction and composite clinical outcome [33].

Summary

The consequences of cardiovascular emergencies in the pregnant patient can be catastrophic and require decisive evaluation, diagnosis, and management in the ED in close consultation with obstetric and surgical colleagues. Initial diagnoses of these life-threatening complications of pregnancy are difficult because symptoms overlap between disease states and with normal pregnancy. Once VTE, aortic dissection, and peripartum cardiomyopathy have been identified, prompt intervention and coordinated interdisciplinary care can make the difference between life and death for both mother and fetus.

Key Points

- Cardiovascular emergencies in pregnancy require prompt recognition, resuscitation, appropriate surgical and obstetrical consultation, and overall coordination of complex interdisciplinary care.
- Signs and symptoms of cardiovascular emergencies significantly overlap with normal physiologic changes and symptoms associated with pregnancy.
- Ionizing radiation exposure to mother and fetus must be considered when selecting an imaging modality; however, a necessary diagnostic test should not be withheld from a pregnant patient out of concern for the fetus.
- Several medications classically used in the treatment of venous thromboembolism, dissection, and cardiomyopathy carry adverse safety profiles in pregnancy and should be avoided.
- Obstetric consultation should be obtained early in the ED course of all pregnant patients with a cardiovascular emergency.

References

1. James A, The Committee on Practice Bulletins. Practice bulletin no. 123: thromboembolism in pregnancy. Obstet Gynecol. 2011;118:718–29.
2. Heit JA, Kobbervig CE, et al. Trends in the incidence of venous thromboembolism during pregnancy or postpartum: a 30-year population-based study. Ann Intern Med. 2005;143(10):697–706.
3. Kamel H, Navi BB, et al. Risk of thrombotic event after the 6-week postpartum period. N Engl J Med. 2014;370(14):1307–15.
4. Conti E, Zezza L, et al. Pulmonary embolism in pregnancy. J Thromb Thrombolysis. 2014;37:251–70.
5. Regitz-Zagrosek V, Lundqvist CB, et al. ESC Guidelines on the management of cardiovascular diseases during pregnancy. Eur Heart J. 2011;32:3147–97.
6. Neggers YH. Trends in maternal mortality in the United States. Reprod Toxicol. 2016;64:72–6. doi:10.1016/j.reprotox.2016.04.001.
7. Van de Pol LM, Mairuhu ATA, Tromeur C, et al. Use of clinical prediction rules and D-dimer tests in the diagnostic management of pregnant patients with suspected acute pulmonary embolism. Blood Rev. 2016; doi:10.1016/j.blre.2016.09.003.
8. Kline JA, Williams GW, Hernandez-Nino J. D-dimer concentrations in normal pregnancy: new diagnostic thresholds are needed. Clin Chem. 2005;51:825–30.
9. Kovac M, Mikovic Z, Rakicevic L, et al. The use of D-dimer with new cutoff can be useful in diagnosis of venous thromboembolism in pregnancy. Eur J Obstet Gynecol Reprod Biol. 2010;148:27–30.
10. Wang M, Lu SM, Li S, et al. Reference intervals of D-dimer during the pregnancy and puerperium period on the STA-R evolution coagulation analyzer. Clin Chim Acta. 2013;425:176–80.

11. Ercan S, Ozkan S, Yucel N, et al. Establishing reference intervals for D-dimer to trimesters. J Matern Fetal Neonatal Med. 2015;28:938–87.
12. Parilla BV, Fournogerakis R, et al. Diagnosing pulmonary embolism in pregnancy: are biomarkers and clinical predictive models useful? Am J Perinatol Rep. 2016;6:e160–4.
13. Chan WS, Chunilal S, Lee A, et al. A red blood cell agglutination D-dimer test to exclude deep venous thrombosis in pregnancy. Ann Intern Med. 2007;147:165–70.
14. Sommerkamp SK, Gibson A. Cardiovascular disasters in pregnancy. Emerg Med Clin North Am. 2012;30:949–59.
15. Leung AN, Bull TM, et al. An official American Thoracic Society/Society of Thoracic Radiology clinical practice guideline: evaluation of suspected pulmonary embolism in pregnancy. Am J Respir Crit Care Med. 2011;184:1200–8.
16. Chagnon I, Bouraneaux H, et al. Comparison of two clinical prediction rules and implicit assessment among patients with suspected pulmonary embolism. Am J Med. 2002;113:269–75.
17. O'Connor C, Moriarty J, et al. The application of a clinical risk stratification score may reduce unnecessary investigations for pulmonary embolism in pregnancy. J Matern Fetal Neonatal Med. 2011;24(12):1461–4.
18. Kline JA, Kabrhel C. Emergency evaluation for pulmonary embolism, part 2: diagnostic approach. J Emerg Med. 2015;49:104–17.
19. Marik PE, Plante LA. Venous thromboembolic disease and pregnancy. N Engl J Med. 2008;359(19):2025–33.
20. Bates SM, Middeldorp S, et al. Guidance for the treatment and prevention of obstetric-associated venous thromboembolism. J Thromb Thrombolysis. 2016;41:92–128.
21. Rajagopalan S, Nwazota N, Chandrasekhar S. Outcomes in pregnant women with acute aortic dissections: a review of the literature from 2003–2013. International Journal of Obstetric Anesthesia. 2014;23:348–56.
22. Poppas A, Shroff SG, et al. Serial assessment of the cardiovascular system in normal pregnancy: role of arterial compliance and pulsatile arterial load. Circulation. 1997;95:2407–15.
23. Nolte JE, Rutherford RB, et al. Arterial dissections associated with pregnancy. J Vasc Surg. 1995;21:515–20.
24. la Chapelle CF, et al. On behalf of the Dutch Maternal Mortality Committee. Maternal mortality attributable to vascular dissection and rupture in the Netherlands: a nationwide confidential enquiry. BJOG. 2012;119:86–93.
25. Sahni G. Chest pain syndromes in pregnancy. Cardiol Clin. 2012;30:343–67.
26. Sliwa K, Hilfiker-Kleiner D, et al. Current state of knowledge on aetiology, diagnosis, management, and therapy of peripartum cardiomyopathy: a position statement from the Heart Failure Association of the European Society of Cardiology Working Group on peripartum cardiomyopathy. Eur J Heart Fail. 2010;12:767–78.
27. Johnson-Coyle L, Jensen L, Sobey A, ACCF AHA. Peripartum cardiomyopathy: review and practice guidelines. Am J Crit Care. 2012;21(2):89–98.
28. Ntusi N, Mayosi B. Aetiology and risk factors of peripartum cardiomyopathy: a systematic review. Int J Cardiol. 2009;131(2):168–79.
29. Elkayam U, Akhter MW, Singh H, Khan S, Bitar F, Hameed A, et al. Pregnancy-associated cardiomyopathy: clinical characteristics and a comparison between early and late presentation. Circulation. 2005;111(16):2050–5.
30. Lampert MB, Lang RM. Peripartum cardiomyopathy. Am Heart J. 1995;130:860–70.
31. Diao M, Diop IB, et al. Electrocardiographic recording of long duration (Holter) of 24 hours during idiopathic cardiomyopathy of the peripartum. Arch Mal Coeur Vaiss. 2004;97:25–30.
32. Lydakis C, Lip GY, Beevers M, Beevers DG. Atenolol and fetal growth in pregnancies complicated by hypertension. Am J Hypertens. 1999;12:541.
33. Sliwa K, Blauwet L, et al. Evaluation of bromocriptine in the treatment of acute severe peripartum cardiomyopathy; a proof-of-concept pilot study. Circulation. 2010;121:1465–73.

Chapter 10
Cardiac Arrest in the Pregnant Patient

Jessica Palmer, Marianne Wallis, and Joelle Borhart

Introduction

Maternal cardiac arrest is among the most stressful and challenging situations an emergency physician can encounter during their career. Two lives are at stake, mother and fetus, and it is generally accepted that the mother's life takes priority in resuscitation, as the best chance for fetal survival is maternal survival. Fortunately, cardiac arrest in pregnancy is rare, complicating an estimated 1 in 12,000 pregnancies in the United States [1]. Maternal mortality is described in the literature as mortality during pregnancy or within 42 days of delivery [2]. Maternal mortality is increasing and was most recently estimated at 15.9 per 100,000 in 2012 [3]. Following cardiac arrest, maternal survival rates range from 17 to 59%, while fetal survival rates range from 61 to 80% depending on the etiology of arrest [4].

The optimal management of maternal cardiac arrest is a multispecialty approach with involvement of emergency physicians, obstetricians, neonatologists, and anesthesiologists. Pregnant patients are a specific population with unique causes of cardiac arrest, and the physiologic changes during pregnancy require distinct modifications during resuscitation.

J. Palmer, M.D. (✉)
Department of Emergency Medicine, MedStar Southern Maryland Hospital,
7503 Surratts Road, Clinton, MD 20735, USA
e-mail: jpalmer1231@gmail.com

M. Wallis, M.D. • J. Borhart, M.D.
Department of Emergency Medicine, MedStar Georgetown University Hospital and MedStar
Washington Hospital Center, 3800 Reservoir Road, NW, Washington, DC 20007, USA
e-mail: mariannewallis@gmail.com; joelle.borhart@gmail.com

© Springer International Publishing AG 2017
J. Borhart (ed.), *Emergency Department Management of Obstetric Complications*,
DOI 10.1007/978-3-319-54410-6_10

Etiologies of Cardiac Arrest

Obstetric Causes

The etiologies of cardiac arrest in the pregnant population can be organized into three groups: obstetrical, non-obstetrical, and iatrogenic (Table 10.1). Obstetric-related etiologies include eclampsia/preeclampsia, amniotic fluid embolism, massive obstetric hemorrhage, and peripartum cardiomyopathy. In developing countries, hemorrhage and eclampsia are the most common [5].

Amniotic fluid embolism, an etiology unique to the pregnant patient, occurs in 1 in 40,000 pregnancies [6]. It is accountable for 10% of peripartum mortality, and maternal mortality rate varies between 20 and 60% [6, 7]. The exact pathophysiology of amniotic fluid embolism is unclear, but current theories are based on the overwhelming maternal inflammatory response to fetal tissue. Initially, disruption of the maternal-fetal barrier, which can occur even in routine labor, leads to release of fetal tissue into maternal circulation. This triggers a brusque maternal inflammatory response, similar to the inflammatory response in anaphylaxis. Indeed, the term "anaphylactoid syndrome of pregnancy" is often used in the literature to describe the condition. Next, a period of uterine hypertonicity leads to fetal distress. Often, it is the signs of fetal distress including late decelerations and fetal bradycardia that are first recognized by providers before maternal signs and symptoms. A consumptive coagulopathy follows, similar to disseminated intravascular coagulopathy.

Amniotic fluid embolism can present as sudden maternal dyspnea and oxygen desaturation during labor or shortly following delivery. Cardiovascular collapse ensues and cardiac arrest is common. Women who survive initial cardiac arrest are prone to acute lung injury and acute respiratory distress syndrome, in addition to anoxic brain injury. Fetal distress occurs along with maternal distress (and may even precede maternal symptoms) as blood is shunted from the uterus to the maternal central circulation for preservation of cardiac and neurologic function.

Treatment for amniotic fluid embolism is primarily supportive. Anoxic brain injury may occur quickly, so a definitive airway should be established early in the resuscitation, and patients should be treated with 100% oxygen [8].

Table 10.1 Causes of cardiac arrest in pregnancy categorized by obstetric, non-obstetric, and iatrogenic etiologies

Causes of cardiac arrest in pregnancy		
Obstetric	Non-obstetric	Iatrogenic
Eclampsia	Pulmonary embolism	General anesthesia-induced
Amniotic fluid embolism	Sepsis	Regional anesthesia-induced
Postpartum hemorrhage	Trauma	Other medications (e.g., magnesium)
Antepartum hemorrhage	Myocardial infarction	Anaphylaxis
Peripartum cardiomyopathy	Aortic dissection	
	Status asthmaticus	
	Anaphylaxis	

Intravascular support in the way of intravenous fluids, blood products, and vasopressors, if necessary, is recommended. Blood products should be considered before clinical signs of hemorrhagic shock. The use of specific factors such as factor VII is not recommended, as these have been linked to vaso-occlusive events [6].

Non-obstetric Causes

Non-obstetric causes of cardiac arrest in pregnancy include sepsis, trauma, myocardial infarction, aortic dissection, anaphylaxis, status asthmaticus, and pulmonary embolism (PE). The most common cause of cardiac arrest in pregnancy in the United States is PE [9]. PE complicates 1 in 1,000 pregnancies, and pregnant women are up to ten times more likely to have a venous thromboembolism than nonpregnant women [10, 11]. When PE is the cause of cardiac arrest, standard advanced cardiac life support (ACLS) therapies are less likely to be effective, necessitating early recognition of this pathology [12]. Clues to PE as the etiology of cardiac arrest include pulseless electrical activity as the initial rhythm as well as a dilated right ventricle on bedside ultrasound [13, 14]. Treatment includes standard ACLS protocol and fibrinolytic therapy. Fibrinolytic options include recombinant tissue plasminogen activators, or synthetic derivatives such as streptokinase and urokinase [15]. A recent meta-analysis of hemodynamically unstable pregnant patients with PE showed the risk of major bleeding following fibrinolysis was low, and the fetal demise rate was only 2.6% [16]. There have been multiple case reports of successful use of fibrinolytic therapy in unstable pregnant women with massive PE, including patients at 26 weeks and 32 weeks with good outcomes [17–19]. Another somewhat novel therapeutic option is extracorporeal membrane oxygenation (ECMO). There have been several case reports showing the use of ECMO for PE with favorable outcomes for both mother and fetus [20, 21].

Iatrogenic Causes

Iatrogenic causes of maternal cardiac arrest include anesthesia-related arrest (both general and regional anesthesia) and medication induced, specifically magnesium toxicity. Anesthesia-induced cardiac arrest is the seventh leading cause of maternal death in the United States [22], although mortality rates are declining [23]. The decline in maternal deaths related to general anesthesia has been attributed to increase the use of pulse oximetry and capnography and utilization of difficult intubation algorithms including the use of supraglottic airway devices. The reduction in maternal deaths from local anesthesia is likely due to using a lower concentration of anesthetics, an increase in general awareness regarding anesthetic toxicity, and an overall emphasis on safety practices [22].

Pregnant patients with systemic anesthetic toxicity present with respiratory and cardiovascular depression, which can eventually lead to complete cardiopulmonary collapse. Treatment is supportive and centered on early recognition, fluid resuscitation, and airway management. Prevention of hypoxia and metabolic acidosis is critical [22]. For patients with complete cardiopulmonary collapse refractory to standard resuscitative measures, lipid emulsion therapy can be considered, though a recent review was inconclusive regarding the efficacy of lipid emulsion therapy for systemic anesthetic toxicity [24].

Another cause of iatrogenic cardiac arrest in pregnancy is magnesium toxicity. Magnesium is a standard therapy for patients with preeclampsia and eclampsia, and there is a risk of cardiopulmonary collapse if toxic levels are reached [25]. Fortunately, toxicity is now rare, as many hospitals have protocols in place to monitor for overdose; however, the possibility still exists and was addressed in recent guidelines from the American Heart Association (AHA) on cardiac arrest [26]. Toxic levels are reached at levels greater than 3.5 mmol/L, although the exact dosing to reach this level is unclear [27]. Symptoms of magnesium toxicity include loss of deep tendon reflexes, respiratory depression, somnolence, and cardiac arrest. If magnesium toxicity is suspected, the infusion should be stopped immediately, and 10 mL of 10% calcium gluconate can be administered [28, 29].

Resuscitation Considerations

ACLS algorithms are generally the same in pregnancy including defibrillation doses and medical management. However, three important differences exist when resuscitating a pregnant patient: (1) positioning of the patient, (2) airway management and anticipation of a difficult airway, and (3) early consideration of perimortem cesarean delivery (PMCD). Additionally, intravenous access should be obtained above the diaphragm in pregnant patients.

Positioning of the Patient

Positioning of a pregnant patient in cardiac arrest is one of the key differences from resuscitating the nonpregnant patient. Once the uterus is palpable above the umbilicus (around 20 weeks), the uterus compresses the aorta and vena cava and decreases venous return when the woman lies supine (aortocaval compression). Chest compressions only produce 30% of normal cardiac output in healthy, nonpregnant patients [30]. In pregnant patients, cardiac output is reduced by an additional 60% in the supine position due to aortocaval compression. Therefore, in pregnant patients, chest compressions in the supine position produce 10% of normal cardiac output at best [31].

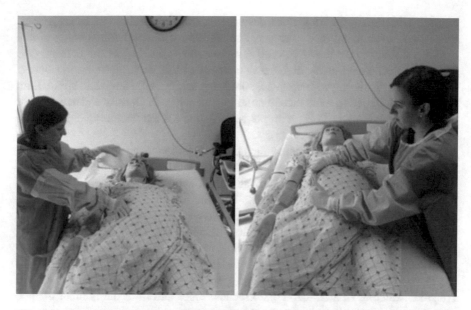

Fig. 10.1 Demonstration of manual uterine displacement on a simulated gravid patient. One-handed approach from the patient's right side, and two-handed approach from patient's left. Note the "pulling" motion of the provider, as opposed to a "pushing" maneuver when using the two-handed approach

Due to aortocaval compression and the resultant limitations on cardiac output, positioning of the pregnant patient is crucial. There are two methods that have been historically used to help decrease aortocaval compression: manual left uterine displacement and lateral tilt. Manual left uterine displacement is the technique currently recommended by the AHA [32]. This can be done using a one-handed technique from the right side of the bed, or with two hands from the left side of the bed (Fig. 10.1a, b). The two-handed approach should be a "pulling" motion instead of a "pushing" motion. Lateral tilt has also been used, although this requires a dedicated foam or wooden wedge and may be less effective [33].

The AHA recommends chest compressions be performed without modifications for the pregnant patient. This includes compressions performed over the lower half of the sternum at a rate of greater than 100 compressions per minute, compressing at a depth of at least 2 in. (5 cm), allowing for complete chest recoil. The compressions to ventilations ratio remains 30 to 2.

Airway Management

Airway management of obstetric patients can be challenging due to anatomical and physiologic changes related to pregnancy. Physiologic changes such as increases in breast tissue and overall weight gain decrease chest wall compliance, making bag-valve-mask ventilation difficult [34]. During late pregnancy, increases in intra-abdominal pressure, a laxity of the lower esophageal sphincter, and slowed gastric emptying increase aspiration risks during endotracheal intubation. In pregnancy, there is an overall increased oxygen demand and decreased functional residual capacity leading to increased susceptibility to hypoxia and rapid desaturation. One study by McClelland et al. in 2009 demonstrated this rapid desaturation during induction of anesthesia, with pregnant subjects reaching SpO2 less than 90% within 5 minutes compared to 9 minutes in nonpregnant subjects. Obesity and active labor accelerate desaturation times, with pregnant patients often becoming significantly hypoxic in less than 3 minutes [35].

Anatomic changes in pregnancy include an overall increase in laryngeal edema. Airway tissue becomes edematous and may prevent the passage of larger (size 7.0 or greater) endotracheal tubes. The Mallampati classification system, historically utilized to evaluate a patient's ability to open their mouth for endotracheal intubation, has been shown to advance one to two classes during pregnancy. These airway changes can persist up to 2–3 weeks following delivery [31].

For all these reasons, emergency physicians should anticipate obstetric patients to be difficult to intubate. Difficult or failed intubation is a major contributory factor to poor maternal outcomes following cardiac arrest [36]. Physicians should consider selecting smaller-sized endotracheal tubes and limit the number of tube passes, as multiple attempts can worsen pre-existing edema. Endotracheal intubation is preferred over supraglottic airways, but laryngeal mask airways (LMAs) and similar adjuncts should be considered following two unsuccessful intubation attempts [32].

Perimortem Cesarean Delivery

Perimortem cesarean delivery (PMCD) describes the procedure of delivering a fetus during maternal cardiac arrest [37]. Historically, the procedure has been performed to potentially benefit the fetus [31]. Over the years, however, it had been observed that when cardiopulmonary resuscitation (CPR) was performed on pregnant patients, return of spontaneous circulation (ROSC) was often achieved after "emptying the uterus" and relieving aortocaval compression [37]. A paradigm shift has since occurred: once considered purely fetocentric, PMCD is now recommended as a primarily maternal resuscitative measure. Indeed, some authors have replaced the term "perimortem cesarean delivery" with "resuscitative hysterotomy" in the literature.

As a general rule, the fundus of the uterus reaches the umbilicus around 20 weeks gestation. It is at this point that the uterus begins to cause significant compression of both the aorta and vena cava, impacting venous return to the maternal heart and increasing maternal afterload [31]. Therefore, any pregnant patient in cardiac arrest with a palpable uterus at, or above, the level of the umbilicus is a candidate for PMCD [4]. Performing the procedure on patients less than 20 weeks gestation is not recommended, as it is not likely to benefit the mother or the fetus.

Anoxic brain injury occurs after 4–6 min of cessation of blood flow. [37] Fetal neurologic sequelae tend to occur later than in the mother following an anoxic event [38]. Historically, PMCD was advised after 4 min of CPR without return of ROSC with the goal of having the baby delivered within 1 minute (the "4-minute rule"). However, this standard can be difficult to attain. A retrospective case review by Benson et al. found 90% of perimortem cesarean deliveries occurred after the 5-minute mark [39]. Additionally, multiple studies have shown positive maternal and fetal outcomes following deliveries well outside the 4-minute window [4, 31, 40]. Some authors recommend performing the procedure immediately in patients with non-shockable rhythms (pulseless electrical activity and asystole) [37]. In patients with ventricular dysrhythmias ("shockable rhythms"), 4 minutes of ACLS prior to PMCD is still advised [41].

Contraindications to PMCD include gestational age less than 20 weeks (or a uterine fundus below the level of the umbilicus in multiple pregnancies), maternal ROSC, and prolonged maternal arrest (typically greater than 15 minutes, although fetal survival has been described in the literature as long as 45 minutes after maternal arrest [42]). Little equipment is needed, and the procedure can be performed with only a scalpel if necessary (Table 10.2). The procedure should be performed by the provider with the most surgical experience, and resuscitation teams for both the mother and fetus should be present.

Table 10.2 Perimortem cesarean section procedure, adapted from Parry R et al. [41]

Procedure: perimortem cesarean section	
Step 1	Preparation • Ensure the patient is supine and continue CPR throughout the procedure • Have resuscitative teams available • Prep the area (if time allows)
Step 2	Skin incision • Vertical midline incision (recommended)—from symphysis pubis to umbilicus dissecting through subcutaneous layer, fascia (white, shiny), and rectus muscles to peritoneum, exposing uterus OR • Horizontal bikini incision—approximately 20 cm in length, two fingerbreadths above the symphysis pubis, dissecting as described above
Step 3	Exposure • Utilize available assistants to retract the abdominal wall, allowing for uterine exposure • Retract the bladder (visualized inferiorly) caudally, to prevent injury
Step 4	Uterine incision • Vertical— midline incision (recommended) make an incision at the lower portion of the uterus extending to the thickened fundus (use scissors if necessary); use the middle and index fingers to lift the uterine wall from the fetus • Horizontal—make an incision approximately 15 cm in length over the thinned lower uterine segment; use the middle and index fingers to lift the uterine wall from the fetus • Cut through the placenta, if needed
Step 5	Delivery • Locate the presenting part through the uterine incision • Apply transthoracic pressure to the uterus while placing traction over the presenting part to deliver the fetus, taking care not to hyperextend the neck of the fetus • Clamp and cut the umbilical cord • Deliver the placenta with steady traction on the umbilical cord or manual removal • Sweep the uterus to ensure complete removal of products

(continued)

Table 10.2 (continued)

Procedure: perimortem cesarean section

Step 6	Uterine recovery and closure
	• Massage the fundus of the uterus to stimulate uterine contraction and limit hemorrhage
	• Give oxytocin 5 units IV
	• Clamp uterine vessels, if actively bleeding
	• Closure
	– If ROSC attained, consider careful, layered closure, if obstetrics available. If not, consider packing the uterus or placing absorbable sutures
	– If ROSC not attained, consider cardiac visualization for direct cardiac massage
	• If actively bleeding, consider additional pharmacological agents, interventional radiology for vessel ligation/embolization, uterine balloon tamponade, or hysterectomy

Post-resuscitation Care

If ROSC occurs, standard post-resuscitative care should be initiated including transfusion of blood products and vasopressor support as needed. Therapeutic hypothermia has shown to be beneficial to neurological outcomes following cardiac arrest in nonpregnant comatose adult patients with ROSC after out-of-hospital cardiac arrest [43]. Data on the use of therapeutic hypothermia in pregnant patients is limited. Case reports suggest it is safe with good outcomes for mother and fetus [44, 45]. Therapeutic hypothermia should be considered on a case-by-case basis in pregnant patients with ROSC following cardiac arrest [30]. If used in pregnancy, the same protocols for postarrest cooling for nonpregnant patients should be used [30, 46].

Extracorporeal membrane oxygenation (ECMO) is a novel therapy for cardiac arrest and can be considered in pregnancy if it is believed that this will increase likelihood of maternal survival [47]. There are multiple case reports supporting its use and demonstrating relative safety for the fetus [48, 49].

Summary

Maternal cardiac arrest is fortunately a rare occurrence in an emergency physician's career. Understanding maternofetal physiology, cardiac arrest etiologies unique to the pregnant patient, and resuscitation modifications is a physician's best preparation. ACLS algorithms in pregnancy are similar to nonpregnant patients with a few unique exceptions including positioning of the patient, anticipation of a difficult airway, and early consideration of PMCD. Therapeutic hypothermia, ECMO, and fibrinolysis can be considered on a case-by-case basis. Following cardiac arrest, the best chance for fetal survival is maternal survival, and interventions should not be withheld from the mother out of concern for the fetus.

Key Points

- ACLS algorithms are generally the same in pregnancy including defibrillation doses and medical management.
- Pregnant patients in cardiac arrest should have their uterus manually displaced to the left.
- Anticipate a difficult airway when intubating an obstetric patient.
- Any pregnant patient in cardiac arrest with a palpable uterus at or above the level of the umbilicus is a candidate for PMCD.
- The best chance for fetal survival is maternal survival; interventions should not be withheld from the mother out of concern for the fetus.

References

1. Mhyre JM, Tsen LC, et al. Cardiac arrest during hospitalization for delivery in the United States, 1998–2011. Anesthesiology. 2014;120(4):810–8.
2. World Health Organization. WHO Maternal mortality ratio (per 100,000 live births). 2016. http://WHO.int/hcalthinfo/statistics/indmaternalmortality/en. Accessed 11 June 2016.
3. Centers for Disease Control and Prevention. Pregnancy mortality surveillance system. 2016. http://www.cdc.gov/reproductivehealth/maternalinfanthealth/pmss.html. Accessed 6 June 2016.
4. Rose CH, et al. Challenging the 4- to 5-minute rule: from perimortem cesarean to resuscitative hysterotomy. Am J Obstet Gynecol. 2015;213(5):653–6.
5. Schneider AP, Nelson DJ, Brown DD. In hospital cardiopulmonary resuscitation: a 30 year review. J Am Board Fam Pract. 1993;6(2):91–101.
6. Clark SL. Clinical expert series: amniotic fluid embolism. Obstet Gynecol. 2014;123:337–48.
7. Kauer K, Bhardwaj M, et al. Amniotic fluid embolism. J Am Clin Pharm. 2016;3(2):153–9.
8. Moore J, Baldisseri M. Amniotic fluid embolism. Crit Care Med. 2005;33(10):S279–85.
9. Atta E, Gardner M. Cardiopulmonary resuscitation in pregnancy. Obstet Gynecol Clin North Am. 2007;34:585–97.
10. Simcox LE, Ormesher E, Tower C, Green IA. Pulmonary thromboembolism in pregnancy: diagnosis and management. Breathe. 2015;11(14):282–9.
11. Anderson BS, et al. The cumulative evidence of venous thromboembolism during pregnancy and puerperium – an 11 year Danish based population-based study of 63,000 pregnancies. Acta Ostetric Gynec Scand. 1998;77:170–3.
12. Logan JK, et al. Evidence based diagnosis and thrombolytic treatment of cardiac arrest or peri arrest due to suspected pulmonary embolism. Am J Emerg Med. 2014;32(7):789–96.
13. Courtney DM, et al. Pulseless electrical activity with witnessed arrest as a predictor of sudden death from massive pulmonary embolism in outpatients. Resuscitation. 2001;49:265–72.
14. Hernandez C, Shuler K, et al. C.A.U.S.E.: cardiac arrest ultra-sound exam—a better approach to managing patients in primary non-arrhythmogenic cardiac arrest. Resuscitation. 2008;76:198–207.
15. Condliffe R, Elliot C, et al. Management dilemmas in acute pulmonary embolism. Thorax. 2013:1–7.
16. Gartman E. The use of thrombolytic therapy in pregnancy. Obstet Med. 2013;6:105–11.
17. Fassulo S, Maringhini G, et al. Thrombolysis for massive pulmonary embolism in pregnancy: a case report. Int J Emerg Med. 2011;4:69.

18. Hall RJC, Young C, Sutton GC, Cambell S. Treatment of acute massive pulmonary embolism with streptokinase during labor and delivery. Br Med J. 1972;4:647–9.
19. GD t R a, LSM R. Treatment options in massive pulmonary embolism during pregnancy; a case-report and review of literature. Thromb Res. 2009;124:1–5.
20. Weinberg L, Kay C, et al. Successful treatment of peripartum massive pulmonary embolism with extracorporeal membrane oxygenation and catheter-directed pulmonary thrombolytic therapy. Anesthes Intensive Care. 2011;39(3):486–91.
21. Bataillard A, Hebrard A, et al. Extracorporeal life support for treatment of massive pulmonary embolism in pregnancy. Perfusion. 2016;31(2):169–71.
22. Suresh MS, Mason CL, Munnur U. Cardiopulmonary resuscitation and the parturient. Best Pract Res Clin Obstet Gynaecol. 2010;24(3):383–400.
23. Hawkins JL, Chang J, et al. Anesthesia-related maternal mortality in the United States: 1979–2002. Obstet Gynecol. 2011;117(1):69–74.
24. Hoegberg LCG, Bania TC, et al. Systematic review of the effect of intravenous lipid emulsion therapy for local anesthetic toxicity. Clin Toxicol. 2016;54(3):167–93.
25. McDonnell MJ, Machatuta NA, Paech MJ. Acute magnesium toxicity in an obstetric patient undergoing general anaesthesia for caesarean delivery. Int J Obstet Anesth. 2010;19(2):226–31.
26. Vanden Hoek TL, Morrison LJ, et al. Part 12: cardiac arrest in special situations: 2010 American Heart Association Guidelines for Cardiopulmonary Resuscitation and Emergency Cardiovascular Care. Circulation. 2010;122:S829–61.
27. Lu JF, Nightingale CH. Magnesium sulfate in eclampsia and preeclampsia pharmacokinetic principles. Clin Pharmacokinet. 2000;38(4):305–14.
28. Olsen-Chen C, Seligman NS. Hypertensive emergencies in pregnancy. Crit Care Clin. 2016;32:29–41.
29. Swartjes JM, Schutte MF, Blecker OP. Management of eclampsia: cardiopulmonary arrest resulting from magnesium sulfate overdose. Eur J Obstet Gynecol Reprod Biol. 1992;47(1):73–5.
30. Berg RA, et al. Part 5: adult basic life support. 2010 American Heart Association Guidelines for Cardiopulmonary Resuscitation and Emergency Cardiovascular Care Science. Circulation. 2010;122:S685–705.
31. Katz VL. Perimortem cesarean delivery: its role in maternal mortality. Semin Perinatol. 2012;36(1):68–72.
32. Jeejeebhoy FM, Zelop CM, et al. Cardiac arrest in pregnancy: a scientific statement from the American Heart Association. Circulation. 2015;32:1747–73.
33. Ip JK, Campbell JP, Bushby D, Yentis SM. Cardiopulmonary resuscitation in the pregnant patient: a manikin based evaluation of methods producing lateral tilt. Anaesthesia. 2013;68:694–9.
34. Biro P. Difficult intubation in pregnancy. Cur Op Anes. 2011;24:249–54.
35. McClelland SH, Bogod DG, Hardman JG. Preoxygenation and apnoea in pregnancy: changes during labour and with obstetric mortality in a computational simulation. Anesthesia. 2009;64:371–7.
36. Donnehy KC, Pian-Smith MC. Airway management of the parturient. Int Anesthesiol Clin. 2000;38(3):147–59.
37. Katz V, Balderston K, DeFreest M. Perimortem cesarean delivery: were our assumptions correct? Am J Obstet Gynecol. 2005;192:1916–21.
38. Baghirzada L, Balki M. Maternal cardiac arrest in a tertiary care centre during 1989–2011: a case series. Can J Anesth. 2013;60(11):1077–84.
39. Benson MD, Padovano A, Bourjelly G, Zhou Y. Maternal collapse: challenging the four-minute rule. EBioMedicine. 2016;6:253–7.
40. Einav S, Kaufman N, Sela HY. Maternal cardiac arrest and perimortem caesarean delivery: evidence or expert-based? Resuscitation. 2012;83(10):1191–200.
41. Parry R, et al. Perimortem caesarean section. Emerg Med J. 2016;33:224–9.

42. Yildirim C, Goksu S, Kocoglu H, et al. Perimortem cesarean delivery following severe maternal penetrating injury. Yonsei Med J. 2004;45:561–3.
43. Benson DW, Williams GR, Spencer FC, Yates AJ. The use of hypothermia after cardiac arrest. Anesth Analg. 1959;38:423–8.
44. Oguagyo K, Oyeteyo O, Stewart D, Costa S, Jones R. Successful use of therapeutic hypothermia in a pregnant patient. Tex Heart Inst J. 2015;42(4):367–71.
45. Chauhan A, Musunuru H, et al. The use of therapeutic hypothermia after cardiac arrest in a pregnant patient. Ann Emerg Med. 2012;60(6):786–9.
46. Scirica BM. Therapeutic hypothermia following arrest. Circulation. 2013;127:244–50.
47. Agerstrand C, Abrams D, et al. Extracorporeal membrane oxygenation for cardiopulmonary failure during pregnancy and postpartum. Ann Thorac Surg. 2016;102(3):774–9.
48. Moore S, Dietl CA, Coleman DM. Extracorporeal life support during pregnancy. J Thorac Cardiovasc Surg. 2016;151(4):1154–60.
49. Leeper RW, Vladis M, Arntfield R, Guo LR. Extracorporeal membrane oxygenation in the acute treatment of cardiovascular collapse immediately post-partum. Interact Cardiovasc Thorac Surg. 2013;17(5):898–9.

Chapter 11
Trauma in Pregnancy

Marcos Mavromaras, Christina Bird, Julie Gorchynski, and Linda Hatch

Introduction

Trauma, specifically motor vehicle collisions (MVC), intimate partner violence (IPV), and falls, represents the majority of non-obstetric fatalities during pregnancy [1, 2]. Seven percent of all pregnancies are affected as a result of trauma [3]. The incidence of trauma increases with gestational age, and over half of traumatic events involving pregnant women occur in the third trimester [3]. While nine out of ten traumatic events in pregnancy are considered minor, 60–70% of fetal losses occur following a minor maternal injury [4]. Pregnancy itself may be considered an independent risk factor for trauma with recent data reporting an increase in IPV among pregnant women [5]. Other risk factors for trauma include younger age (<25 years), substance or alcohol use, improper use of seatbelts, and low maternal educational or socioeconomic level [6–9]. MVC comprise approximately 50% of all traumas in pregnancy with IPV and falls comprising approximately 22% [1, 3, 10–12].

Emergency physicians often evaluate pregnant women after minor and serious trauma. An understanding of the anatomical and physiological changes during pregnancy as well as injuries unique to the pregnant patient is critical. The optimal management of the pregnant trauma patient involves a multidisciplinary team of emergency physicians, obstetricians, trauma surgeons, and neonatologists. Emergency physicians are in a unique position to educate pregnant patients on injury prevention including proper seatbelt use as well as screen for IPV.

M. Mavromaras, M.D. • C. Bird, D.O. (✉) • J. Gorchynski, M.D. • L. Hatch, M.D.
Department of Emergency Medicine, UT Health Science Center,
MC7736, 7703 Floyd Curl Drive, San Antonio, TX 78229, USA
e-mail: mavromaras@uthscsa.edu; birdc@uthscsa.edu; gorchynski@uthscsa.edu

© Springer International Publishing AG 2017
J. Borhart (ed.), *Emergency Department Management of Obstetric Complications*,
DOI 10.1007/978-3-319-54410-6_11

Common Mechanisms of Trauma in Pregnancy

Motor Vehicle Collisions

Motor vehicle collisions are the leading cause of trauma in pregnancy, and 82% of traumatic fetal deaths occur following an MVC. Lack of seatbelt use or incorrect belt placement increases the risk of intrauterine injury and fetal death and is the major risk factor for adverse outcomes following MVC [4, 13]. Indeed, unrestrained pregnant women in MVC are twice as likely to have preterm delivery within 48 h and 2.8 times more likely to experience a fetal death than if they were appropriately restrained [14, 15]. Compliance with seatbelt usage and proper placement of seatbelts are decreased in pregnant women. There is a false impression that seatbelts "will hurt the baby." Pregnant women often incorrectly position restraints, which make the restraints less effective in preventing injury to both mother and fetus. Three-point restraint should include the shoulder strap resting between the breasts and around gravid abdomen, while the lap portion should rest snugly over the hips below the gravid abdomen [16]. Higher level of education appears to correlate with increased seatbelt usage among this population [17]. Emergency physicians should educate and encourage pregnant patients regarding diligent usage and proper placement of seatbelts.

Intimate Partner Violence

One in five teens and one in six adult women experience IPV during pregnancy, amounting to approximately 335,000 cases in the United States annually [18]. Risk factors associated with IPV during pregnancy include substance abuse, witnessed domestic violence as a child, low maternal educational or socioeconomic level, unplanned pregnancy, history of prior IPV, and unmarried status [19]. IPV may occur for the first time during pregnancy, or the severity of violence may escalate [20]. Pregnant victims of IPV are at risk for both immediate- and long-term sequelae such as placental abruption, uterine rupture, prematurity, and low birth weight infants, respectively, resulting in maternal and fetal mortality [18, 21, 22]. Since 2013, the US Preventive Services Task Force has recommended screening of all women of childbearing age for IPV in the emergency department (ED).

Falls

Pregnant women are at higher risk of falling as gait is affected by weight gain and increased joint laxity and postural stability is decreased. Indeed, one in four women will fall during the course of their pregnancy [13]. Most falls occur indoors, and 39% are associated with stairs [23]. Falls often result in orthopedic injuries, with fractures of the lower extremities being most common [24]. Isolated orthopedic injuries place the pregnant patient at significantly higher risk for adverse obstetric outcomes including preterm birth, placental abruption, low birth weight infants, and increased perinatal mortality. Additionally, there is a ninefold increased risk of thrombotic events following orthopedic injury [10]. For these reasons, emergency physicians should have a low threshold for observing and monitoring pregnant patients after even minor isolated orthopedic injuries.

Anatomic and Physiologic Considerations in Pregnancy

The uterus is relatively protected within the pelvis until between 8 and 12 weeks after which it starts to ascend, reaching the level of the umbilicus at approximately 20 weeks [25]. The ascending and enlarging uterus displaces the intestine and stomach upward, changing the location of abdominal pain. From the second trimester forward, the peritoneum may be less irritable due to the peritoneum and abdominal musculature being stretched from the gravid uterus [26]. There can be significant trauma within the pelvis and abdomen without peritoneal signs [27]. The unreliability of the abdominal exam may lead to delayed diagnoses of internal injuries [28]. Between 8 and 12 weeks, the bladder also ascends slightly into the abdomen, itself becoming more susceptible to injury. The diaphragm may be up to 4 cm higher than in a nonpregnant patient, which, on imaging, may cause an apparent widened mediastinum, enlarged cardiac silhouette, and decreased lung volumes. Additionally, this may result in a left axis shift and flattened T waves on ECG (Fig. 11.1).

Emergency Department Evaluation and Management

Primary Survey

The general principles of Advanced Trauma Life Support (ATLS) apply to all pregnant trauma patients, with a few exceptions. The first priority of management of the pregnant trauma patient is to attend to the mother. Optimal care of the mother amounts to optimal fetal care. The ED evaluation of the pregnant trauma patient begins with a rapid and thorough assessment of the mother with simultaneous initiation of IV crystalloids, supplemental oxygen, and left lateral decubitus positioning to avoid hypotension. Vital signs in pregnant trauma patients are unique in that pregnant women normally have relative tachycardia, hypotension, and tachypnea due to physiological changes of pregnancy.

Early recognition of pregnancy is critical in the trauma patient. All women of childbearing age presenting with trauma should have a pregnancy test performed. In one study, 8% of pregnant women that were admitted to a trauma center were unaware they were pregnant [29]. The abdomen should be palpated for a gravid uterus. It is widely accepted that a clinical estimation of gestational age of ≥24 weeks, which correlates with a fundal height of 3–4 finger breaths above the umbilicus, corresponds to a potentially viable fetus and an increased likelihood of extrauterine survival [27].

Successful management of the pregnant trauma patient requires a multidisciplinary approach including a trauma surgeon, obstetrician, and neonatologist

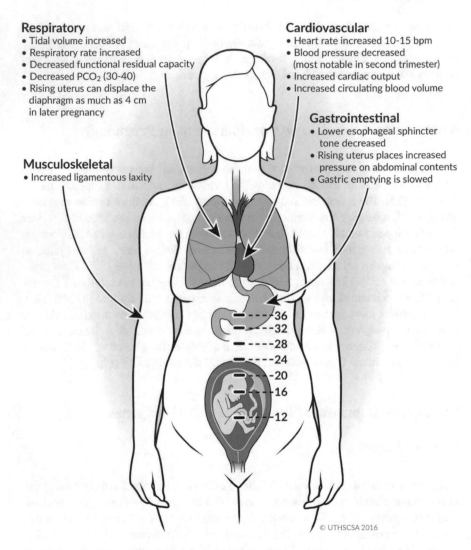

Respiratory
- Tidal volume increased
- Respiratory rate increased
- Decreased functional residual capacity
- Decreased PCO_2 (30-40)
- Rising uterus can displace the diaphragm as much as 4 cm in later pregnancy

Cardiovascular
- Heart rate increased 10-15 bpm
- Blood pressure decreased (most notable in second trimester)
- Increased cardiac output
- Increased circulating blood volume

Gastrointestinal
- Lower esophageal sphincter tone decreased
- Rising uterus places increased pressure on abdominal contents
- Gastric emptying is slowed

Musculoskeletal
- Increased ligamentous laxity

36
32
28
24
20
16
12

© UTHSCSA 2016

Fig. 11.1 Anatomic and Physiologic Considerations of Pregnancy

working in conjunction with the emergency physician. The emergency physician must weigh the resources available at their facility and be prepared to mobilize and coordinate other resources if they should become necessary. Many minor trauma patients present to non-trauma centers, and even innocuous appearing injuries may have potentially life-threatening implications to the fetus or mother. Therefore, transfer to a trauma center or a facility that has continuous fetal cardiotocographic monitoring capabilities is strongly encouraged.

Airway

Due to the risk of fetal hypoxia, early airway management is highly recommended in caring for the pregnant trauma patient, especially if the patient is obtunded or displaying signs of respiratory compromise [25]. The emergency physician should have a low threshold for intubation and mechanical ventilation and anticipate a difficult airway [30].

Intubation failure rate has been reported to be higher in pregnant patients due to the various anatomical and physiological changes that occur in pregnancy. Diaphragmatic elevation decreases forced vital capacity. The relative hypocapnia of pregnancy, together with a baseline decrease in functional residual capacity and residual volume, results in decreased oxygen reserves. There is a propensity toward faster desaturation during rapid sequence intubation (RSI); therefore preoxygenation is vital [31–35]. Normal pregnancy causes fluid retention and weight gain resulting in mucosal edema and therefore narrower airways. This also increases airway resistance and decreases overall respiratory system compliance. Endotracheal tubes with diameters 0.5–1.0 mm smaller than standard tube sizes should be used on the first attempt, with smaller tubes prepared as backup [36]. In addition, there is increased aspiration risk during intubation for the pregnant trauma patient due to the ascending and enlarging uterus which places increased pressure on intestinal and stomach contents; at the same time progesterone-mediated smooth muscle relaxation reduces the tone of the lower esophageal sphincter [37, 38]. A low threshold for the placement of a nasogastric tube for gastric decompression prior to RSI is recommended.

The majority of RSI medications, including paralytics, analgesics, anesthetics, or sedatives, are category C under the FDA pregnancy pharmacology safety guidelines (Table 11.1). Exceptions include ketamine, which is category B, and benzodiazepines that are category D (Table 11.2). There are no current recommendations or guidelines to suggest the use of one medication over another or dose adjustments for RSI in the pregnant patient [31–33].

Breathing

If mechanical ventilation is initiated, minute ventilation should be managed to maintain $PaCO_2$ levels around 30–32 mm Hg, as hypocapnia is physiologic in late pregnancy. A $PaCO_2$ >32 mmHg in a pregnant patient suggests respiratory insufficiency and a level >40 mmHg, respiratory failure [30]. Fetal survival is entirely dependent upon uterine perfusion and oxygen delivery.

Avoidance of an acidotic state is essential as it is thought to result in uterine vasoconstriction [34].

Targets of SaO2 > 95% and PaO2 > 70 mm Hg ensure fetal oxygen delivery; PaO2 < 60 mmHg has been associated with compromise of fetal oxygenation [28, 35, 37, 39]. In the event of a pneumo–/hemothorax, the chest tube should be placed 1–2 interspaces higher due to diaphragmatic elevation in order to avoid entering the abdomen [25].

Table 11.1 FDA drug risk classification in pregnancy[a]

Category	Description
A	Controlled studies in humans show no risk to the fetus
B	Animal studies show no risk to the fetus, no controlled studies in humans
C	No controlled studies in animals or humans
D	Evidence of human risk to the fetus exists; however benefits may outweigh risks
X	Controlled studies demonstrate fetal abnormalities. Risk outweighs any possible benefit

[a]As of 2014 the FDA is changing drug labeling regarding its use during pregnancy or lactation and phasing out the letter categories [61]

Table 11.2 Safety profiles of commonly used medications

Category	Medications	Safety profile
Paralytics	Rocuronium	B
	Succinylcholine	C
	Vecuronium	C
Analgesics/sedatives	Ketamine	B
	Propofol	B
	Opiates	C
	Benzodiazapines	D
	Dexmedetomidine	C
Vasopressors	All	C
Antiemetics	Ondansetron	B
	Metoclopramide	B
	Phenothiazines	C
	Pyridoxine (vitamin B6)	A

Circulation

Plasma blood volume steadily increases throughout pregnancy; therefore a pregnant patient may lose up to 2 L of blood before showing any signs of circulatory instability [25]. Cardiac output is also increased and can result in rapid hemorrhage. Serum HCO3 < 19 may be an early indication of circulatory compromise.

In the event of hemorrhage, the fetus is at risk for reduced blood supply because maternal circulation preferentially shunts blood away from the uterus. Furthermore, uterine compression of abdominal and pelvic vasculature after 20-week gestation can result in decreased venous return and resultant "supine hypotensive syndrome." Patients should be placed in the left lateral decubitus position when possible or the uterus should be manually displaced to the left of the midline [26, 40, 41]. Angulations of the patient on the backboard to achieve a slight left lateral decubitus position of 15° to 30° or right lateral decubitus positioning are acceptable alternatives [30, 40]. Intravenous (IV) access, whether central or peripheral, should be established above the level of the diaphragm due to possible uterine compression of abdominal and pelvic vasculature [30].

When treating a pregnant trauma patient, the clinician should avoid the pitfall of attributing hypotension to supine hypotensive syndrome and should ensure that the patient is not hemorrhaging. Recommendations on resuscitative blood pressure goals are extrapolated from perioperative cesarean section patients. The American Heart Association (AHA) recommends a goal for systolic blood pressure (SBP) of >100 mm Hg or greater than 80% of the patient's baseline blood pressure [42]. Alternatively, the mean arterial pressure (MAP) can be targeted to a value of >65 mmHg as extrapolated from studies in nonpregnant patients. In order to maintain uterine perfusion, hypotension should be aggressively managed. Urinary output is the most sensitive prognosticator of maternal cardiovascular collapse [43]. It is recommended that early requisition and utilization of blood products, specifically CMV antibody-negative or leukocyte-reduced, Rh-negative products, must be transfused in a 2:1:1 (red blood cell/plasma/platelets) ratio given the relative hemodilution in pregnant women [44]. Vasopressors may reduce uterine flow and therefore placental perfusion, but the benefits of correcting maternal hemodynamics are of primary concern. The preferential use of phenylephrine has increased in popularity due to recent studies demonstrating less hypotension and improved fetal acid-base status compared to the once previously utilized ephedrine [45].

Secondary Survey

The secondary survey should proceed according to ATLS guidelines in the same fashion as nonpregnant women with the addition of fetal heart rate monitoring initiated in the ED if available. Patients who suffer direct abdominal trauma or who present with contractions, vaginal bleeding, or uterine tenderness are more likely to have obstetric complications [46]. All pregnant women should have a sterile bimanual exam performed to evaluate for the presence of the fetus, fetal body parts, umbilical cord, placenta, or uterus within the vaginal vault and to determine if any disruption of the rectal and vaginal mucosa has occurred. The clinician should also assess for ruptured membranes or acute vaginal hemorrhage. Any of these findings require immediate surgical and obstetric consultations for imminent fetal delivery in a more controlled environment. Placental abruption, uterine rupture, and preterm labor may occur following even minor abdominal trauma [3, 25]. Bedside focused assessment of sonography in trauma (FAST) can determine the presence of free fluid, pneumothorax, hemothorax, pericardial effusion, and uterine rupture, if present. In the rare event that diagnostic peritoneal lavage is performed, a supraumbilical open approach is recommended to avoid inadvertent uterine injury.

Uterine contractions are the most common presenting obstetric symptoms after abdominal trauma and are usually self-limited [27]. The identification of pathologic contractions is important as they may have deleterious effects on the fetus. Tocolysis may be necessary depending on the gestational age of the fetus in consultation with an obstetrician. Terbutaline 0.25 mg subcutaneous is recommended as the first-line agent and intravenous magnesium as an adjunct [25]. If the fetus is between 24 and 34 weeks, corticosteroids and betamethasone 12 mg or dexamethasone 6 mg intramuscular (IM) should be given to promote fetal lung maturity if delivery seems probable [25].

Diagnostic Studies

Laboratory Tests

Initial laboratory tests include pregnancy test, complete blood count (CBC), complete metabolic panel (CMP), coagulation studies, lactate, and blood type and cross match. Because plasma volume increases during pregnancy, a mild decrease in hematocrit is physiologic; however, in the setting of trauma, there is always the possibility of ongoing blood loss. Standard parameters for lab values such as CMP, coagulation studies, and lactate are largely unchanged in the pregnant trauma population. Specific predictors of fetal hypoxia include a decrease in hematocrit of greater than 50%, PaO_2 <60 mmHg (O_2 sat<90%), as well as acidosis. Increased minute ventilation and tidal volume result in a relative hypocapnia and respiratory alkalosis with baseline $PaCO_2$ of 30 mmHg; a $PaCO_2$ of 40 mmHg indicates CO_2 retention. However, serum pH can generally normalize due to renal compensation.

Type and cross match with Rh status should be included in a basic trauma lab set. Reportedly, as little as 0.001 mL of fetal blood in the maternal circulation can sensitize an Rh-negative mother [47]. Therefore rhesus immune globulin (RhIG) should be administered to all Rh-negative mothers following even minor trauma. In the first trimester, one 50 mcg intramuscular dose is sufficient prophylaxis. In the second and third trimesters, 300 mcg is needed to provide prophylaxis for up to 30 mL of fetal-maternal hemorrhage. There is no harm in giving the more readily available 300 mcg dose to women in the first trimester. The Kleihauer-Betke (KB) quantifies the amount of fetal-maternal hemorrhage, and KB analysis may have a role in directing the obstetrician in administering additional doses of RhIG in small subset of women where fetal-maternal hemorrhage may be in excess of 30 mL [3]. The results of the KB test will not impact ED care. Some literature reports higher rates of preterm labor in patients with a positive KB test [48]. Flow cytometric assay has been useful in quantifying fetal-maternal hemorrhage in preference to the KB technique [49]. The initial dose of RhIG prevents Rh isoimmunization up to 72 h following antigenic exposure.

Imaging

Decisions regarding imaging in pregnant trauma patients are often fraught with apprehension. The potential risk associated with ionizing radiation exposure to the fetus should be considered when obtaining imaging studies; however maternal resuscitation is of primary concern. A necessary diagnostic test should not be withheld out of concern for the fetus. Radiation harm to the fetus and risk of teratogenesis is greatest during the 8th through the 15th week of gestation when organogenesis occurs [10] (Table 11.3). Exposure to ionizing radiation doses above 100–200 mGy is associated with intrauterine growth retardation and CNS defects, such as microcephaly and mental retardation. Ionizing radiation doses less than 50 mGy have not been associated with difference in overall pregnancy outcomes. The fetal dose without shielding is approximately 30% of that to the mother [3]. Redundant imaging should be avoided, for example, if a patient is getting computed tomography (CT) scans of the abdomen and pelvis, and then the pelvic x-ray may not be necessary [3].

Ultrasound carries no risk of ionizing radiation and is considered safe during pregnancy [50]. M-mode imaging should be used instead of spectral Doppler imaging to document fetal heart rate [50]. FAST scan is an effective modality to identify free intra-abdominal fluid with greater than 90% specificity but with 61% sensitivity [51]. Chest and pelvic x-rays are the more commonly ordered images in trauma. Chest X-ray should be done with abdominal shielding in known pregnant patients. Most X-rays are considered very low-dose examinations and pose almost no risk to the fetus [52]. While CT studies confer the most radiation risk, the studies most commonly used in trauma evaluation expose the fetus to ionizing radiation doses well below 50 mGy [53] (Table 11.4). Magnetic resonance imaging (MRI) is considered safe in pregnancy; however gadolinium is contraindicated due to possible teratogenic effects [53]. Often in trauma, time is of the essence and MRI may not be practical.

Table 11.3 Effects of gestational age and radiation dose on radiation-induced teratogenesis

Gestational period	Effects	Estimated threshold dose[a]
Before implantation (0–2 weeks after conception)	Death of embryo or no consequence (all or none)	50–100 mGy
Organogenesis (2–8 weeks after conception)	Congenital anomalies (skeleton, eyes, genitals)	200 mGy
	Growth retardation	200–250 mGy
Fetal period		
8–15 Weeks	Severe mental retardation (high risk)[b]	60–310 mGy
	Intellectual deficit	25 IQ point loss per gray
	Microcephaly	200 mGy
16–25 Weeks	Severe mental retardation (low risk)	250–280 mGy

[a]Data based on results of animal studies, epidemiologic studies of survivors of the atomic bombings in Japan, and studies of groups exposed to radiation for medical reasons (e.g. radiation therapy for carcinoma of the uterus)
[b]Because this is a period of rapid neuronal development and migration
Patel S J, Reede D L, Katz D S, et al. Imaging the pregnant patient for nonobstetric conditions: Algorithms and radiation dose considerations. RadioGraphics 2007;27:1705–1722. With permission

Traumatic Injuries Specific to the Pregnant Patient

Abruptio Placenta

Abruption occurs when the placenta becomes separated from the uterine wall and is most commonly due to shearing forces related to trauma. Abruption has been reported to occur in up to 2–4% of even minor trauma. Patients may present with abdominal or pelvic pain with or without vaginal bleeding. The clinical signs and symptoms may be subtle. The amount of vaginal bleeding does not necessarily reflect the severity of the abruption, as a large hemorrhage can be concealed behind the placenta. Abruptions of less than 50% commonly result in fetal distress. Fetal demise almost always occurs in the event of greater than 50% abruption unless the fetus can be immediately delivered [27]. In patients beyond 24 weeks, continuous cardiotocodynamometry is the most sensitive predictor of abruption after trauma [25]. In one study, all cases of placental abruption showed frequent contractions, more than eight per hour, in the initial 4 h of electronic fetal monitoring [54]. Ultrasound has a sensitivity of 24% and 96% specificity [22, 49, 55]. Therefore, a negative ultrasound cannot exclude placental abruption. When positive, ultrasound shows retroplacental hemorrhage that is hyperechoic. Lab values such as elevated D-dimer, decreased fibrinogen, and elevated fibrin split products are associated with abruption but are neither sensitive nor specific [25].

Table 11.4 Fetal radiation doses associated with common radiological axaminations

Type of examination	Fetal absorbed dose[a] (mGy)
Very low-dose examinations (<0.1 mGy)	
• Cervical spine X-ray (AP and lateral)	<0.001
• Any extremity X-ray	<0.001
• Chest X-ray (two views)	0.0005–0.01
Low- to moderate-dose examinations (0–10 mGy)	
Radiography	
• Thoracic spine X-ray	0.003
• Abdominal X-ray	0.1–3
• Lumbar spine X-ray	1–10
• Intravenous pyelography	5–10
• Double-contrast barium enema	1–20
CT	
• Head, neck, or extremity[b]	0–10
• Chest CT or CT pulmonary angiography	0.01–0.66
Nuclear medicine	
• Low-dose perfusion scintigraphy	0.1–0.5
• V/Q scintigraphy	0.1–0.8
Higher-dose examinations (10–50 mGy)	
• Abdominal CT	1.3–35
• Pelvic CT	10–50
• Abdomen and pelvis	13–25
• Aortic angiography of chest, abdomen, pelvis with or without contrast agent	6.7–56
• Coronary artery angiography	0.1–3
• Nonenhanced CT of abdomen and pelvis to evaluate for nephrolithiasis	10–11

CT computed tomography, *V/Q* ventilation/perfusion
[a]Fetal dose varies with gestational age, maternal body habitus, and exact acquisition parameters
[b]Most authors report fetal dose from the head, neck, or extremity CT close to zero (negligible scatter)

Uterine Rupture

Uterine rupture is rare, estimated to complicate only 0.6% of traumatic injury [48]. Risk factors include multiparty, prior uterine surgery, polyhydramnios, and multiple gestations [49, 56]. Fetal mortality approaches 100% and maternal mortality 10% [27]. A loss of palpable uterine contour as well as palpation fetal parts may be found on physical exam, and ultrasound may show abnormal fetal location.

Amniotic Fluid Embolism

Amniotic fluid emboli may occur in the setting of even minor trauma including all types of blunt trauma injuries [10, 57]. Symptoms are rapidly progressive and include disseminated intravascular coagulation, acute respiratory failure, and cardiac arrest. Treatment is largely supportive. Pulmonary vasodilators such as inhaled nitric oxide, sildenafil, and prostacyclin may have theoretical benefit in moving the emboli through the lungs, but lack any significant evidence [10].

CardioPulmonary Arrest and Perimortem Cesarean Delivery

In the event of acute cardiopulmonary arrest in the pregnant patient whose uterus extends beyond the umbilicus, maternal survival requires uterine-aortocaval decompression. This may be accomplished by performing a perimortem cesarean delivery (PMCD). Delivery of the fetus aides in maternal survival by decreasing aortocaval compression, increasing venous return to the heart, and increasing cardiac output by 60–80% [58]. Indeed, some authors advocate using the term "resuscitative hysterotomy" to describe the procedure to emphasize the maternal benefits [59]. The most experienced physician should perform PMCD, and cardiopulmonary resuscitation (CPR) should be continued during the procedure. Obtaining fetal heart tones is not required prior to performing a PMCD. Ideally, the fetus should be delivered within 4–5 min from the initiation of CPR, although there are reports of positive maternal and fetal outcomes beyond this recommendation [60]. Favorable fetal-maternal outcomes are linked to earlier PMCD; however, the procedure is often unnecessarily delayed. The placenta must be removed from the uterus following delivery of the infant to maximize cardiac output. Closure of the uterus, fascia, peritoneum, and skin may be delayed until the return of spontaneous circulation is achieved [2]. Fear of litigation may hinder the clinician from performing a PMCD; however, there are no reported cases of litigation against an emergency physician for having performed a PMCD.

Disposition

Fetal compromise may not be apparent during the initial evaluation in the ED. Continuous cardiotocodynamometry should be performed in pregnant trauma patients presenting ≥24-week gestation for at least 4 h following even minor trauma [26]. If there is any question of fetal viability, the clinician should err on the side of performing continuous fetal heart monitoring until dates can be confirmed by ultrasound or other techniques [30]. In the event that there is no supportive obstetric care on-site, the patient should be transferred to a facility capable of providing continuous cardiotocodynamic monitoring and obstetric intervention. Criteria for admission and operative indications are otherwise similar for pregnant and nonpregnant trauma patients.

Summary

Trauma in pregnancy is a critically important topic for the emergency physician. It is the unique situation of caring for two patients simultaneously. Efficient and vigilant care of the mother takes precedence and generally ensures better outcomes for both mother and fetus. Motor vehicle collisions, intimate partner violence, and falls are the most common mechanisms of trauma encountered. The emergency physician should seek to have a firm understanding of the specific anatomical and physiological changes of the pregnant patient as outlined above to ensure optimum care for their patients. The care of a pregnant patient in a trauma situation should include a multidisciplinary approach involving trauma surgeons and obstetricians early in the resuscitation. Emergency physicians are encouraged to err on the side of continuous monitoring or transfer to a facility capable of such in the event of a viable fetus with concern or question of potential injury.

Key Points

- The mother takes priority during the trauma resuscitation.
- A pregnancy test should be obtained in all female trauma patients of childbearing age.
- Motor vehicle collisions, intimate partner violence, and falls represent the majority of non-obstetric fatalities during pregnancy.
- Unrestrained pregnant women have higher rates of complications including preterm labor and fetal death. Emergency physicians should educate pregnant patients about appropriate use of three-point restraint.
- Relative tachycardia, hypotension, and tachypnea make it more difficult to identify hemodynamic instability early.
- Perimortem cesarean delivery should be performed within 4 min of initiation of CPR when possible.
- Pregnant patients with a viable fetus should have continuous cardiotocodynamic monitoring for at least 4 h following even minor trauma.

References

1. El-Kady D, Gilbert WM, Anderson J, et al. Trauma during pregnancy: an analysis of maternal and fetal outcomes in a large population. Am J Obstet Gynecol. 2004;190(6):1661–8.
2. Fildes J, Reed L, Jones N, et al. Trauma: the leading cause of maternal death. J Trauma. 1992;32(5):643.
3. Barraco R, Chiu WC, Clancy T, et al. Practice management guidelines for the diagnosis and management of injury in the pregnant patient: the EAST Practice Management Guidelines Work Group. J Trauma. 2010;69:211–4.
4. Murphy NJ, Quinlan JD. Trauma in pregnancy: assessment, management, and prevention. Am Fam Physician. 2014;90:717–22.
5. Gazmararian JA, Lazorick S, Spitz AM, et al. Prevalence of violence against pregnant women. JAMA. 1996;275:1915–20.
6. Weiss HB. Pregnancy-associated injury hospitalizations in Pennsylvania, 1995. Ann Emerg Med. 1999;34(5):626–36.
7. McFarlane J, Parker B, Soeken K, et al. Assessing for abuse during pregnancy. Severity and frequency of injuries and associated entry into prenatal care. JAMA. 1992;267(23):3176–8.
8. Stewart D, Cecutti A. Physical abuse in pregnancy. CMAJ. 1993;149:1257–63.

9. Helton AS, McFarlane J, Anderson ET. Battered and pregnant: a prevalence study. Am J Public Health. 1987;77:1337–9.
10. Smith K, Bryce S. Trauma in the pregnant patient: an evidence-based approach to management. Emerg Med Pract. 2013;15(4).
11. Weiss H, Songer TJ, Fabio A. Fetal deaths related to maternal injury. JAMA. 2001;286(15):1863–8.
12. Chang J, Berg CJ, Saltzman L, et al. Homicide: a leading cause of injury deaths among pregnant and postpartum women in the United States, 1991–1999. Am J Public Health. 2005;95(3):471.
13. Mendez-Figueroa H, Dahlke JD, Vrees Ram et al. Trauma in pregnancy: an updated systematic review. Am J Obstet Gynecol. 2013;209:1–10.
14. Hyde LK, Cook LJ, Olson LM, et al. Effect of motor vehicle crashes on adverse fetal outcomes. Obstet Gynecol. 2003;102(2):279–86.
15. Wolf ME, Alexander BH, Rivara FP, et al. A retrospective cohort study of seatbelt use and pregnancy outcome after a motor vehicle crash. J Trauma Injury Infect Crit Care. 1993;34:116–9.
16. Berghella V. Maternal-Fetal evidence based guidelines. 2nd ed. CRC Press; 2011. p. 276–84.
17. Sirin H, Weiss HB, Sauber-Schatz EK, et al. Seat belt use, counseling and motor-vehicle injury during pregnancy: results from a multi-state population-based survey. Matern Child Health J. 2007;11(5):505–10.
18. Parker B, McFarlane J, Soeken K. Abuse during pregnancy: effects on maternal complications and birth weight in adult and teenage women. Obstet Gynecol. 1994;84:323–8.
19. Umeora OU, Dimejesi BI, et al. Pattern and determinants of domestic violence among prenatal clinic attendees in a referral center, south-east Nigeria. J Obstet Gynaecol. 2008;28:769–74.
20. American College of Obstetricians and Gynecologists. Intimate partner violence. ACOG Committee Opinion No. 518. Obstet Gynecol. 2012;119:412–7.
21. El Kady D, Gilbert WM, Xing G, et al. Maternal and neonatal outcomes of assaults during pregnancy. Obstet Gynecol. 2005;105(2):357–63.
22. Leone JM, Lane SD, Koumans EH, et al. Effects of intimate partner violence on pregnancy trauma and placental abruption. J Womens Health. 2010;19(8):1501–9.
23. Dunning K, Lemasters G, Bhattacharya A. A major public health issue: the high incidence of falls during pregnancy. Matern Child Health J. 2010;14:720–5.
24. Schiff MA. Pregnancy outcomes following hospitalization for fall in Washington state from 1987 to 2004. BJOG. 2008;115:1648–54.
25. Tibbles. Trauma in pregnancy: double jeopardy. Emerg Med Pract. 2008;10(7).
26. Chames MC, Pearlman MD. Trauma during pregnancy: outcomes and clinical management. Clin Obstet Gynecol. 2008;51(2):398–408.
27. Hanley M, Thomson C. Trauma in pregnancy: double jeopardy. Emerg Med Pract 2003:5(1).
28. Catanzarite V, Willms D, Wong D, et al. Acute respiratory distress syndrome in pregnancy and the puerperium: causes, courses, and outcomes. Obstet Gynecol. 2001;97(5):760–4.
29. Bochicchio GV, Napolitano LM, Haan J, et al. Incidental pregnancy in trauma patients. J Am Coll Surg. 2001;192:566–9.
30. Mallemat H. Supportive management of critical illness in the pregnant patient. EM Crit Care. 2012;2(3).
31. Hawkins JL, Arens JF, Bucklin BA, et al. Practice guidelines for obstetric anesthesia: an updated report by the American Society of Anesthesiologists Task Force on Obstetric Anesthesia. Anesthesiology. 2007;106(4):843–63.
32. Bergen JM, Smith DC. A review of etomidate for rapid sequence intubation in the emergency department. J Emerg Med. 1997;15(2):221–30.
33. Lutes M, Slawter A. Focus on: emergency airway management in the pregnant patient, in ACEP News. 2007. ACEP.
34. Lapinsky SE, Kruczynski K, Slutsky AS. Critical care in the pregnant patient. Am J Respir Crit Care Med. 1995;152(2):427–55.
35. Tomimatsu T, Pereyra Peña JL, Longo LD. Fetal cerebral oxygenation: the role of maternal hyperoxia with supplemental CO_2 in sheep. Am J Obstet Gynecol. 2007;196(4):359e1–5.
36. Izci B, Vennelle M, Liston WA, et al. Sleep-disordered breathing and upper airway size in pregnancy and post-partum. Eur Respir J. 2006;27(2):321–7.

37. Hill CC, Pickinpaugh J. Physiologic changes in pregnancy. Surg Clin North Am. 2008;88(2):391–401.
38. Chestnutt A. Physiology of normal pregnancy. Crit Care Clin. 2004;20(4):609–15.
39. Tomimatsu T, Pereyra Pena J, Hatran DP, et al. Maternal oxygen administration and fetal cerebral oxygenation: studies on near-term fetal lambs at both low and high altitude. Am J Obstet Gynecol. 2006;195(2):535–41.
40. Ellington C, Katz VL, Watson WJ, et al. The effect of lateral tilt on maternal and fetal hemodynamic variables. Obstet Gynecol. 1991;77(2):201–3.
41. Kundra P, Khanna S, Habeebullah S, et al. Manual displacement of the uterus during caesarean section. Anaesthesia. 2007;62(5):460–5.
42. Vanden Hoek TL, Morrison LJ, Shuster M, et al. Part 12: cardiac arrest in special situations: 2010 American Heart Association guidelines for cardiopulmonary resuscitation and emergency cardiovascular care. Circulation. 2010;122(18):S829–61.
43. Roemer K. Becerra O, et al. Trauma in the obstetric patient: a bedside tool https://www.acep.org/Clinical---Practice-Management/Trauma-in-the-Obstetric-Patient--A-Bedside-Tool/.
44. Socol ML, Flint PT. ACOG practice bulletin Prevention of Rh D alloimmunization. Int J Gynecol Obstet. 1999;66:63–70.
45. Habib A. A review of the impact of phenylephrine administration on maternal hemodynamics and maternal and neonatal outcomes in women undergoing cesarean delivery under spinal anesthesia. Anesth Analg. 2012;114(2):377–90.
46. Clinical policy: critical issues in the initial evaluation and management of patients presenting to the emergency department in early pregnancy. Ann Emerg Med. 2003;41: 123–33.
47. Jain V, Chari R, Maslovitz S, et al. Guidelines for the management of a pregnant trauma patient. J Obstet Gynaecol Can. 2015;37:553–71.
48. Muench MV, Baschat AA, Reddy UM, et al. Kleihauer-Betke testing is important in all cases of maternal trauma. J Trauma. 2004;57(5):1094–8.
49. Carey JL, McCoy JP, Keren DF. Flow cytometry in clinical diagnosis. 2007:11.
50. Doubilet PM, Benson CB. First, do no harm ... to early pregnancies. J Ultrasound Med 2010. 29: p. 685–689.
51. Richards JR, Ormsby EL, Romo MV, et al. Blunt abdominal injury in the pregnant patient: detection with US. Radiology. 2004;233(2):463–70.
52. American College of Obstetricians and Gynecologists Committee on Obstetric Practice Committee Opinion 656: guidelines for diagnostic imaging during pregnancy and lactation. Practice Obstet Gynecol. 2016;127:e75–80.
53. Wang PI, Chong ST, Kielar AZ, et al. Imaging of pregnant and lactating patients: part 1, evidence-based review and recommendations. Am J Roentgenol. 2012;198(4):778–84.
54. Pearlman MD, Tintinalli J, Lorenz RP. A prospective controlled study of outcome after trauma during pregnancy. Am J Obstet Gynecol. 1990;162:1502–10.
55. Dijkman A, Huisman CMA, Smit M, et al. Cardiac arrest in pregnancy: increasing use of perimortem caesarean section due to emergency skills training? BJOG. 2010;117(3):282–7.
56. Jeejeebhoy FM, et al. Cardiac arrest in pregnancy: a scientific statement from the American Heart Association. Circulation. 2015;132:1747–73.
57. Ellingsen CL, Eggebø TM, Lexow K. Amniotic fluid embolism after blunt abdominal trauma. Resuscitation. 2007;75(1):180–3.
58. Hill CC, Pickinpaugh J. Trauma and surgical emergencies inthe obstetric patient. Surg Clin North Am. 2008;88(2):421–40.
59. Rose CH, Faksh A, Traynor KD, et al. Challenging the 4-5 minute rule: from perimortem cesarean to resuscitative hysterotomy. Am J Obstet Gynecol. 2015;213:653–6.
60. Jeejeebhoy FM, Zelop CM, Windrim R, et al. Management of cardiac arrest in pregnancy: a systematic review. Resuscitation. 2011;87(7):801–9.
61. Content and format of labeling for human prescription drug and biological products; requirements for pregnancy and lactation labeling. Food and Drug Administration. December 2014. https://federalregister.gov/a/2014-28241.

Chapter 12
Non-obstetric Abdominal Pain in Pregnancy

Mallory Shasteen and Elizabeth Pontius

Introduction

Abdominal pain in pregnancy has a wide differential diagnosis, and many of the causes are unrelated to the pregnancy itself. As many as 1 in 500 pregnant women develop an acute abdomen, and up to 1% of women need an operation during pregnancy for a non-obstetric problem [1, 2]. Anatomic and physiologic changes in pregnancy put the pregnant woman at an increased risk for certain conditions. Additionally, diagnosing the cause of abdominal pain in pregnancy may be challenging. The gravid uterus may displace abdominal organs, peritonitis may not develop due to abdominal musculature stretching, and leukocytosis is unreliable due to leukocytosis of pregnancy. These changes, along with a hesitancy to perform radiographic tests in pregnant women, can make it difficult to determine the diagnosis and subsequently lead to a delay in treatment. This chapter discusses the causes, presentation, diagnosis, and management of non-obstetric abdominal pain that can occur in pregnant women, ranging from gynecologic to genitourinary to gastrointestinal (Table 12.1).

M. Shasteen, M.D.
Department of Emergency Medicine, Greenville Hospital System, 4 Majestic Oak Court, Greenville, SC 29609, USA
e-mail: mallory.shasteen@gmail.com

E. Pontius, M.D., R.D.M.S. (✉)
Department of Emergency Medicine, MedStar Washington Hospital Center, 110 Irving Street NW, Washington, DC 20010, USA
e-mail: epontius@gmail.com

© Springer International Publishing AG 2017
J. Borhart (ed.), *Emergency Department Management of Obstetric Complications*,
DOI 10.1007/978-3-319-54410-6_12

Table 12.1 Non-obstetric causes of abdominal pain in pregnancy

Gynecologic	Genitourinary	Gastrointestinal
Ovarian torsion	Urinary tract infection	Appendicitis
Ovarian cysts	Pyelonephritis	Cholelithiasis/cholecystitis
Fibroids	Urolithiasis	Pancreatitis
Round ligament pain	–	Diverticulosis/diverticulitis
Vaginal infections	–	Bowel obstruction
Pelvic inflammatory disease	–	Inflammatory bowel disease
–	–	GERD/peptic ulcer disease
–	–	Constipation

Appendicitis

Appendicitis is the most common cause of non-obstetric emergency surgery in pregnancy, affecting 1 of every 1500 pregnancies and accounting for approximately one-quarter of non-obstetric operations [1, 2, 4]. The incidence of appendicitis in pregnant women is the same as the incidence of appendicitis in nonpregnant women, with 40% of cases occurring in the second trimester [1, 2]. Appendix rupture is two to four times more common in pregnant women than nonpregnant women, often due to diagnostic delay or hesitancy to perform an operation [1, 2, 5]. A perforated appendix increases fetal mortality from 0–1.5% to 20–35% [1, 2].

Diagnosing appendicitis in pregnancy can be challenging. The clinical presentation of appendicitis during pregnancy may differ from that of nonpregnant women, especially in the third trimester when the growing uterus can displace the appendix cranially and pain may be felt in the right flank or right upper quadrant [2, 6, 7]. Computed tomography (CT) is commonly used in nonpregnant patients to diagnose appendicitis, but should be used judiciously during pregnancy. Ultrasound and magnetic resonance imaging (MRI) are alternative imaging modalities that are safe during pregnancy [1]. A sequential imaging approach may be necessary. Ultrasound is more readily available, less expensive, and easier to perform; however, if ultrasound is inconclusive, MRI without contrast may be useful to rule out appendicitis due to its higher sensitivity (33–100% for ultrasound versus 80–100% for MRI) [8–10]. In addition, MRI may also reveal alternative causes of the patient's abdominal pain, such as ovarian masses, intra-abdominal abscess, and nephrolithiasis [11]. If MRI is inconclusive, unavailable, or impractical, CT may be performed in consultation with obstetricians, radiologists, and the patient. The risks associated with a missed diagnosis of acute appendicitis are high and generally considered to outweigh the risks of radiation to the fetus [12, 13]. A necessary diagnostic test should not be withheld from a pregnant patient out of concern for the fetus.

Appendicitis is a surgical emergency, and delayed treatment leads to increased maternal complications, including septic shock, peritonitis, and venous thromboembolism, as well as increased fetal loss [1, 2, 4]. Delaying operative intervention may also lead to increased fetal morbidity, including preterm delivery and fetal loss [14]. In remote areas where surgical services are not available, intravenous antibiotic therapy should be used as a bridge during transport to a higher level of care [15].

Cholelithiasis/Cholecystitis

Increased estrogen levels during pregnancy lead to increased cholesterol formation, and higher progesterone levels during pregnancy slow movement of the gallbladder and lead to bile stasis. When combined, these lead to increased development of cholelithiasis and cholecystitis [1, 16, 17]. Symptomatic gallstone disease affects 0.05–3% of pregnancies, and cholecystitis is the second most common non-obstetric surgical complication during pregnancy, affecting approximately 0.1% of pregnancies [1, 2, 13, 16]. The signs and symptoms of gallbladder disease in pregnant women are similar to those in their nonpregnant counterparts: nausea, vomiting, fever, right upper quadrant or epigastric pain radiating to the back, and symptoms that worsen with eating [1].

Ultrasound is the diagnostic test of choice for gallstone disease and cholecystitis [1]. If concern exists for choledocholithiasis, endoscopic retrograde cholangiopancreatography (ERCP) should be performed as it is both diagnostic and therapeutic. Magnetic resonance cholangiopancreatography (MRCP) can be performed prior to ERCP; however, MRCP may miss small stones less than 6 mm [18].

Patients with symptomatic cholelithiasis or cholecystitis may be treated surgically or conservatively with hydration, antibiotics, symptom control, and delayed cholecystectomy after pregnancy is complete [1]. However, conservative treatment of symptomatic cholelithiasis leads to higher symptom recurrence rate, increases the number of emergency department (ED) visits and hospitalizations, and increases the incidence of both cholecystitis and biliary pancreatitis [2, 13, 16, 19]. Rates of spontaneous abortions vary from 0 to 12% with conservative management and 0–2% with surgical management [16, 20].

Pancreatitis

Acute pancreatitis in pregnancy is rare, affecting less than 0.05% of pregnancies, with more than 50% of cases occurring in the third trimester [1, 21]. Symptoms are similar to those in nonpregnant women: pain, nausea, vomiting, and fever [1]. Gallstone disease is the most common cause of pancreatitis in pregnancy, occurring in about two-thirds of patients, but elevated triglyceride levels may also cause pancreatitis. Rarely, preeclampsia can cause vascular change in the pancreas as well [1, 13, 21, 22].

Management of pancreatitis includes hydration, bowel rest, and analgesia, with early resumption of enteral feeding [1, 22]. Feeding should begin by the mouth after symptom resolution in mild acute pancreatitis or by nasogastric tube in severe pancreatitis. Total parental nutrition should be avoided in pregnancy, as pregnant patients are at higher risk of acquiring catheter-related infections [24]. Recurrent gallstone pancreatitis occurs in 70% of pregnant patients, compared with 20–30% of the general population; thus, surgical consultation for cholecystectomy planning should be considered during the first episode [13, 22].

Abdominal ultrasound can be used to look for a dilated common bile duct, cholelithiasis, pancreatic abscess, and pancreatic pseudocysts; MRI also provides excellent soft tissue imaging and can be used to look for complications [1]. Endoscopic ultrasound, ERCP, and MRCP can also aid in the evaluation for common bile duct stones and should be considered if symptoms of moderate to severe pancreatitis do not improve after 2–3 days of treatment [22–24].

Due to advances in diagnosis and treatment, maternal mortality from pancreatitis has decreased from 30 to 40% in the 1970s to less than 1% in the 2000s [22]. Fetal loss secondary to maternal pancreatitis has decreased significantly as well, from near 50% to less than 5%, but can be as high as 20% when acute pancreatitis occurs in the first trimester [23, 25–27].

Diverticulosis/Diverticulitis

Diverticular disease is typically a disease of elderly patients; thus it often is forgotten in the differential diagnosis of abdominal pain in pregnancy. However, there are case reports of diverticulitis with perforation as the ultimate cause of a pregnant patient's abdominal pain [28], and incidence of diverticular disease at one facility was 1 in 600 pregnancies [5]. Symptoms of diverticulitis may mimic that of appendicitis if the condition is right sided or due to a Meckel's diverticulitis [28, 29]. Imaging with ultrasound, MRI, or CT should be considered to help differentiate the cause of the patient's pain [5, 28]. Treatment with antibiotics may remove the need for surgical intervention; however, if surgery is required, a laparoscopic approach is recommended [5, 29].

Bowel Obstruction

As many as 1 in 1500 pregnancies are complicated by bowel obstruction [1, 12, 30]. Maternal mortality is as high as 6%, but can reach 20% in the third trimester; fetal mortality can be as high as 26% [1]. Bowel obstructions can be due to adhesions, either secondary to prior surgery or pelvic inflammatory disease, intussusception, hernias, or carcinoma. Additionally, the rapidly growing uterus can cause mechanical compression of the gastrointestinal tract; thus bowel obstruction is most common in the third trimester when the uterus is at its largest [1, 12]. In pregnant patients, volvulus is a common cause of bowel obstruction, found in 25–44% of obstructed patients, unlike in the general population where the incidence is much lower (<1%) [3, 12, 30].

Symptoms of bowel obstruction are nonspecific, as many women experience abdominal distension, pain, nausea, vomiting, and constipation as part of pregnancy [3]. Diagnosis of volvulus can often be made by plain radiograph, with a characteristic horseshoe-shaped distended bowel loop seen in 80–90% of cases. In other cases, ultrasound, MRI, colonoscopy, or even CT may be required to make the diagnosis [3, 30, 31]. Bowel obstruction may respond to conservative therapy (bowel rest, nasogastric suction, fluid and electrolyte replacement), but many cases require operative intervention, especially if signs of bowel necrosis, perforation, or peritonitis are present [3, 12, 30, 32, 33]. Occasionally, endoscopy or flexible sigmoidoscopy can successfully reduce a volvulus, allowing for operative intervention after completion of pregnancy [34, 35].

Inflammatory Bowel Disease

Inflammatory bowel disease (IBD) encompasses both ulcerative colitis (UC) and Crohn's disease (CD). If the disease is inactive at conception, approximately one-third of patients experience a relapse during pregnancy, most often during the first trimester or immediate postpartum period. If conception occurs during active disease, disease activity persists or worsens in two-thirds of patients [5, 36]. Disease activity at conception and throughout pregnancy is associated with higher rates of spontaneous abortion, preterm delivery, and low birth weight infants [37–39]. Pregnancy complications, including preeclampsia, preterm premature rupture of membranes, and venous thromboembolism, are higher in patients with IBD [39].

Symptoms of IBD flares include abdominal pain, diarrhea, rectal bleeding, and weight loss. Evaluation is similar to that of nonpregnant patients; however, laboratory testing should include testing stool for *Clostridium difficile*, as this is more common in pregnancy [40]. If imaging studies are necessary, MRI without contrast is preferred to CT scanning, to limit radiation exposure to the fetus. Flexible sigmoidoscopy and colonoscopy can also be used to investigate disease severity [40, 41].

Treatment of IBD typically involves a combination of aminosalicylates, corticosteroids or other immune suppressants, and antibiotics [5]. The aminosalicylates, sulfasalazine, and mesalazine are considered safe to use in pregnancy, though women should receive 2 mg of daily folic acid supplementation to prevent folate deficiency [5, 37, 39, 41, 42]. In animal studies, corticosteroids have led to a higher rate of spontaneous abortions, low birth weight, and cleft palate; however, these studies have not been validated in humans [5, 37, 40, 42]. Corticosteroid use is associated with gestational diabetes, low birth weight, and preterm birth [39]. Thus, corticosteroids should be used at the lowest effective dose and for the shortest duration possible [5, 37, 39, 40]. The decision to use azathioprine, 6-mercaptopurine, infliximab, and cyclosporine, though generally considered to be safe in pregnancy, should be made in consultation with both gastroenterology and obstetrics colleagues [5, 37, 38, 40]. The use of methotrexate is contraindicated in pregnancy, as it is a known teratogen [5, 37, 39–42]. Metronidazole and quinolones are the antibiotics used most commonly to treat flares of IBD in nonpregnant patients. Some human studies have shown increased rates of cleft lip and cleft palate with the use of metronidazole; thus, its use should be avoided in the first trimester [39–42]. Most authors agree that quinolones should be avoided during pregnancy due to cartilage toxicity shown in animal studies, though no harm has been shown in human case reports [5, 37, 39–42]. Macrolide antibiotics and amoxicillin-clavulanic acid can be used as alternatives [5, 39, 40].

Pregnant women with Crohn's disease may be at higher risk of surgical complications of CD than nonpregnant women with CD, particularly anorectal abscesses and intestinal-genitourinary fistulas [36]. Indications for surgery in IBD include severe bleeding, disease refractory to medical management, perforation, obstruction, and abscess [39, 40, 42]. Surgical intervention for IBD during pregnancy has led to increased rates of spontaneous abortion and stillbirth [5].

Gastroesophageal Reflux Disease and Peptic Ulcer Disease

Gastroesophageal reflux disease (GERD) affects 30–85% of women during pregnancy, and symptoms typically worsen during pregnancy for those women already diagnosed with GERD [37, 43, 44]. The growing uterus increases intra-abdominal pressure, and increased estrogen and progesterone levels during pregnancy lead to lower esophageal sphincter relaxation and decreased gastrointestinal motility. Symptoms include heartburn, nausea, vomiting, regurgitation, epigastric pain, anorexia, dysphagia, water brash, chronic cough, and sore throat [43, 44]. Symptoms may worsen after meals or when lying flat [37, 43].

Treatment begins with diet and lifestyle modifications; however, if these are not successful, antacids and sucralfate are safe to use in pregnancy [37, 43, 44]. Histamine type 2 receptor antagonists are likely safe in pregnancy, but proton pump inhibitors should be used only in refractory cases, as some animal studies have shown teratogenic effects [37, 43–45], The pro-motility agent metoclopramide is safe in pregnancy and can improve GERD symptoms by promoting gastric emptying and increasing lower esophageal sphincter pressure [44].

Ulcer development and perforation can occur during pregnancy, though perforation is rare [45]. Ulcer perforation causes acute severe abdominal pain, nausea, and vomiting. Peritoneal signs such as guarding, rebound, and tense abdominal wall should prompt surgical evaluation [45, 46].

Constipation

Constipation is a common complaint during pregnancy, affecting as many as 40% of women [5, 44, 47]. Patients present with abdominal pain, bloating, and occasionally with blood in the stool after straining [44]. Causes include increased levels of estrogen and progesterone which increase bowel transit time, mechanical blockage from the growing uterus, decreased level of maternal activity, as well as iron supplementation common during pregnancy [5, 43, 44].

Treatment focuses on patient education, with the goal of increasing dietary water and fiber intake and maternal exercise. Bulking agents and probiotics may also be helpful, and stool softeners are safe to use in pregnancy [5, 43, 44, 48, 49]. Osmotic and stimulant laxatives such as sorbitol can be used when other measures fail but can lead to electrolyte disturbances, so should only be used for short duration [5, 43, 44]. Mineral oil, castor oil, and saline hyperosmotic agents should be avoided in pregnancy, as they may lead to neonatal hypoprothrombinemia and hemorrhage, uterine contractions, and maternal fluid retention, respectively [44].

Ovarian Torsion

Pregnancy is a risk factor for ovarian torsion, though torsion occurs rarely affecting 1 in 5000 pregnancies [50, 51]. Torsion may involve the ovary, fallopian tube, or both [52]. It is caused by partial or complete twisting of the vascular pedicle, which leads to venous, arterial, and lymphatic obstruction that can ultimately result in ovarian necrosis [52]. When ovarian torsion occurs during pregnancy, it usually occurs in the first trimester—this is most likely due to the higher incidence of functional cysts during this period [50, 51]. Ovarian torsion is more common on the right side due to the longer right ovarian ligament, which results in increased mobility of the right ovary. The presence of the sigmoid colon in the left adnexa decreases the mobility of the left ovary [50, 51]. In addition to pregnancy, risk factors for ovarian torsion include increased ovarian size, ovarian tumors, and ovarian hyperstimulation. Assisted reproductive treatments and ovarian hyperstimulation may increase the size of ovaries and subsequently increase the chance of adnexal torsion [50]. The incidence of ovarian torsion rises to 6% after ovarian stimulation and up to 16% in cases of ovarian hyperstimulation syndrome [51]. An ovarian mass 6–8 cm is most likely to undergo torsion [50].

The most common symptom of ovarian torsion is lower abdominal pain [52, 53]. Other presenting signs and symptoms include nausea, vomiting, fever, adnexal mass, and leukocytosis [50, 51, 53]. These symptoms are nonspecific which can lead to misdiagnosis, delayed treatment, and complications such as loss of a fallopian tube or ovary [51, 53]. Pelvic ultrasound with Doppler is the imaging modality of choice, and the most common finding is an enlarged ovary or an echoic adnexal mass [50, 52–54]. The absence of arterial and venous blood flow has a 94% positive predictive value for ovarian torsion and is predictive of a nonviable ovary [52, 54]. Pelvic ultrasound with Doppler flow, however, has a high false-negative rate for ovarian torsion because of the dual blood supply from the ovarian artery and the utero-ovarian vessels [54]. The presence of blood flow on Doppler ultrasound does not rule out ovarian torsion. Early diagnosis and prompt surgical intervention are critical in order to preserve the pregnancy and the patient's fertility [50, 53].

Laparoscopic surgery in early pregnancy has been shown to be safe for the fetus and is preferable to laparotomy [50, 51]. Delay in surgery may lead to serious infection and jeopardize the lives of both the fetus and mother [50].

Adnexal Masses and Ovarian Cysts

The incidence of adnexal masses during pregnancy ranges between 0.2 and 2% [55, 56]. The majority of adnexal masses are found incidentally during first trimester ultrasound, but 1–2% become symptomatic during the first trimester and can develop complications that require surgical intervention [55]. The most common adnexal masses during pregnancy are functional cysts, such as follicular cysts and corpus luteal cysts, which are hormonally influenced [56, 57]. Functional cysts typically resolve spontaneously after the first 14–16 weeks of gestation. Other causes of adnexal mass during pregnancy include dermoid cysts, serous and mucinous cystadenomas, and endometriomas, which are all benign tumors [55, 56].

Ovarian cysts in pregnancy most commonly occur during the first trimester. Cysts may become symptomatic due to rupture, hemorrhage, or torsion. The main presenting symptom is acute abdominal pain, with or without signs of hemodynamic instability. Pelvic ultrasound (transabdominal or transvaginal) is used to diagnose ruptured or hemorrhagic ovarian cysts [57]. If the ultrasound diagnosis is uncertain or an adnexal mass is too big to fully assess by ultrasound, non-contrast MRI can be used. Gadolinium-based contrast material should be avoided in pregnancy [56].

Most ovarian cysts in pregnancy will resolve spontaneously. Surgical intervention is required in the case of suspected ovarian torsion. Although most adnexal masses during pregnancy are benign, ectopic and heterotopic pregnancy should be ruled out in patients who present with a symptomatic adnexal mass early in pregnancy.

Fibroids

Uterine fibroids, or leiomyomas, are benign smooth muscle tumors of the uterus. Approximately 20–50% of women of reproductive age have fibroids, and the incidence of fibroids increases with maternal age at pregnancy [58, 59]. During pregnancy, the size of fibroids can fluctuate. The majority does not significantly change in size, but one-third of fibroids may grow in the first trimester. The larger the size of the fibroid, the higher the risk is of adverse events in pregnancy [58, 60, 61].

Most fibroids are asymptomatic in pregnancy, but they can lead to complications including miscarriage, hemorrhage, abdominal pain, preterm labor, malposition of the fetus, red degeneration, retained products of conception, and intrauterine growth restriction (IUGR). The most common complications in order of frequency are abdominal pain (47%), threatened preterm labor, and anemia. Painful fibroids in pregnancy are most often seen in women with large fibroids (>5 cm) during the second and third trimesters of pregnancy. Pain is usually due to "red degeneration," which is the result of decreased blood supply to the fibroid causing the fibroid to turn red and become necrotic [57–61]. Rupture, hemorrhage, and acute twisting of fibroids also cause pain.

Fibroids and their complications can often be diagnosed and evaluated by pelvic ultrasound [59, 61]. Treatment for painful fibroids is primarily conservative. Rarely, opioid analgesia or surgical management is required for patients who do not respond to conservative management [58, 60]. Surgical management via myomectomy during pregnancy is reserved for cases of severe intractable pain as the risks include severe hemorrhage, pregnancy injury, and pregnancy loss [59].

Round Ligament Pain

Round ligament pain is caused by physiologic changes that occur as the uterus increases in size during pregnancy. The round ligament suspends the uterus in place, and as the uterus grows, the ligaments stretch and can cause pain. Presenting symptoms are pelvic pain and low back pain. Symptoms are usually worse on the right side because the uterus tends to turn to the right. The pain occurs suddenly, often after changing positions or at night, and can be severe. Round ligament pain is a diagnosis of exclusion. Treatment is conservative and includes frequent rest, hot and cold compresses, supportive belts, acupuncture, and yoga [57].

Urinary Tract Infections and Pyelonephritis

Urinary tract infections (UTI) in pregnancy can be divided into three categories: asymptomatic bacteriuria, cystitis, and pyelonephritis. Asymptomatic bacteriuria is defined as $>10^5$ CFU/ml in midstream clean-catch specimens or $>10^2$ CFU/ml in catheterized urine specimens. The prevalence of asymptomatic bacteriuria is between 5 and 10% of pregnancies [63]. Physiologic changes in pregnancy including reduction in smooth muscle tone, slowing of ureteral peristalsis, and compression of the bladder leading to vesicoureteral reflux and urine retention promote ascending infections and make the pregnant woman with asymptomatic bacteriuria more susceptible to development of cystitis and pyelonephritis [62, 63]. For this reason, asymptomatic bacteriuria in pregnant women should be treated. In randomized controlled trials, treatment of pregnant women with asymptomatic bacteriuria has been shown to decrease the incidence of pyelonephritis, preterm birth, and low birth weight infants [64]. Twenty to thirty percent of pregnant women with asymptomatic bacteriuria can progress to pyelonephritis if left untreated [62, 63].

Cystitis is defined as the presence of small bacterial colony counts in the setting of cloudy urine, dysuria, frequency, urgency, abdominal pain, or suprapubic pain [63]. Urine culture remains the gold standard for diagnosing UTI but is not necessary in most cases of uncomplicated infections. Urinalysis with >10 leukocytes per HPF or with positive leukocyte esterase and/or nitrates can be used to diagnose UTI in the emergency department [62].

Acute pyelonephritis is evidence of UTI via urinalysis (>10 WBC and <2–4 epithelial cells) or urine culture (>10^5 CFU/ml) in addition to at least one of the following: fever, flank pain, or costovertebral angle tenderness [65]. The prevalence of acute pyelonephritis is between 0.5 and 2% of pregnancies. Pyelonephritis is most common in late pregnancy, with 80–90% of cases occurring in the second and third trimesters. Risk factors for pyelonephritis include asymptomatic bacteriuria, maternal age, nulliparity, sickle cell anemia, diabetes, nephrolithiasis, illicit drug use, history of pyelonephritis, and maternal urinary tract defects [63].

The most common pathogens responsible for UTI during pregnancy are similar to those in nonpregnant women: *E. coli*, *Klebsiella pneumoniae*, coagulase-negative *Staphylococcus*, *S. aureus*, and group B streptococci. Nearly all antimicrobials cross the placenta and some can cause teratogenic effects. The use of fluoroquinolones is contraindicated throughout pregnancy due to the effect on fetal cartilage development. Aminoglycosides and tetracyclines also have teratogenic effects and should be avoided during pregnancy if possible. Trimethoprim-sulfamethoxazole should be avoided in the first trimester [63]. Ampicillin and amoxicillin should be avoided in the treatment of UTI due to the high rate of resistance [65]. Antimicrobial selection for the treatment of asymptomatic bacteriuria and cystitis is similar (Table 12.2), but cystitis requires a longer duration of antibiotics. Treatment of cystitis and pyelonephritis should be initiated before the results of the urine culture are available if culture was ordered [64].

Hospital admission is recommended for pregnant patient with pyelonephritis for the initial 48 h of treatment, and parenteral antibiotics continued until the patient is no longer febrile. Parenteral antibiotics should be initiated empirically based on clinical evidence, then tailored based on culture results. Once the patient is afebrile for 48 h, she can be switched to oral antibiotics to be continued for 10–14 days [63]. Additional testing in cases of pyelonephritis includes complete blood count, basic metabolic panel, and ultrasound of the kidneys to exclude renal abscess, ureter obstruction, and other abdominal infections.

Kidney Stones

The incidence of kidney stones, or urolithiasis, is the same in pregnant women as in nonpregnant women, affecting 1:200–1:2500 pregnancies [66]. Kidney stones are most common during the second half of pregnancy, with 80–90% of kidney stones in pregnant women occurring in the second and third trimester [67]. Patients present most commonly with flank pain and hematuria. Other symptoms can include nausea, vomiting, fevers, chills, and dysuria. The diagnosis can be challenging as pregnancy-induced hydronephrosis can cause flank pain that can mimic urolithiasis [68]. Ultrasound is considered the first-line imaging modality, but is limited by the low and variable sensitivity (34–94%) and specificity (72–97%). MRI has a specificity of 80%, but may not be readily available. Ultralow-dose CT is an alternative imaging modality with sensitivity of 97% and specificity of 95%, but should be reserved for rare cases as there is no long-term safety data [66].

Initial treatment of kidney stones is conservative (IV fluids and analgesia), as 50–80% of pregnant women will pass the stones spontaneously [66, 67]. Surgical intervention is required if there is persistent obstruction or intractable pain. A kidney stone in the setting of pyelonephritis can result in urosepsis and premature labor. These patients may require temporary treatment with nephrostomy, stenting, or definitive ureteroscopy. A study by Adanur et al. found that semirigid ureteros-

Table 12.2 Antibiotic regimens for asymptomatic bacteriuria, cystitis, and pyelonephritis in pregnancy

	Antibiotic	Dose	Duration	Notes
Asymptomatic bacteriuria	Cephalexin	500 mg PO q6-12 h	3–7 days	
	Amoxicillin/ clavulanic acid	500 mg PO q8h or 875 mg PO q12h	3–7 days	
	Nitrofurantoin	100 mg PO q12h	5–7 days	Contraindicated 38–42 weeks gestation (risk of hemolytic anemia)
	Cefpodoxime	100 mg PO q12h	3–7 days	
	Fosfomycin	3 g PO	Single dose	
Acute cystitis	Cephalexin	500 mg PO q6h	7–14 days	
	Amoxicillin/ clavulanic acid	500 mg PO q8h or 875 mg PO q12h	7–14 days	
	Nitrofurantoin	100 mg PO q12h	7–14 days	Contraindicated 38–42 weeks gestation (risk of hemolytic anemia)
	Cefpodoxime	100 mg PO q12h	7–14 days	
	Fosfomycin	3 g PO	Single dose	
Pyelonephritis	Ceftriaxone	1 g IV q24h		
	Cefepime	1 g IV q12h		
	Aztreonam	1 g IV q8h		
	Ampicillin plus gentamicin	1–2 g IV q6h 1.5 mg/kg IV q8h		

copy is safe for treatment of pregnant patients with refractory symptomatic stones that cannot pass spontaneously [67].

Pelvic Inflammatory Disease

Pelvic inflammatory disease (PID) is a polymicrobial infection-induced inflammation that involves the upper female genital tract including the endometrium, fallopian tubes, ovaries, and peritoneum. It is caused by spontaneous ascension of microorganism from the cervix or vagina [69]. PID includes endometritis, salpingitis, tubo-ovarian abscess, and pelvic peritonitis [70]. Acute PID during pregnancy is rare, but most often occurs in the first trimester before the cervical mucous plug can act as an adequate barrier [71]. Symptoms can include mucopurulent vaginal discharge, pelvic pain, nausea, vomiting, diarrhea, and fever. Findings on pelvic exam include cervical motion tenderness, uterine tenderness, and adnexal tenderness, and at least one must be present to make the diagnosis. Leukocytosis and leukocyturia can also be present in acute PID [54, 69, 71]. Acute PID may be mistaken for appendicitis.

The etiology of PID is polymicrobial: *N. gonorrhoeae*, *C. trachomatis*, *M. genitalium*, and aerobic/anaerobic bacteria that are endogenous vaginal flora [70]. The most common organism cultured from patients with PID is *N. gonorrhoeae* [72]. Bacterial vaginosis (BV) is frequently present in women with PID; one study found that two-thirds of women with PID had BV [70].

Treatment includes antimicrobials that provide coverage of all the potential organisms, even if screening for *N. gonorrhoeae* and *C. trachomatis* is negative as this does not rule out upper genital tract infection with these organisms [69]. Treatment of acute PID can prevent long-term sequelae such as infertility, ectopic pregnancy, and chronic pelvic pain. Administration of empiric antibiotics within 72 h helps to prevent long-term sequelae and should, therefore, be started as soon as the presumptive diagnosis is made. Pregnant women with PID are at high risk for maternal morbidity and preterm delivery; for this reason they should be hospitalized and treated with parenteral antibiotics. Inpatient regimens include cefotetan 2 g IV q12h + doxycycline 100 mg PO or IV q12h, cefoxitin 2 g IV q6h + doxycycline 100 mg PO or IV q12h, or clindamycin 900 mg IV q8hr + gentamicin 3–5 mg/kg IV daily [69, 70]. Due to the potential teratogenic effects of doxycycline, azithromycin can be substituted as a 500 mg IV single dose followed by azithromycin 250 mg PO daily. Parenteral therapy can be discontinued 24–48 h after the patient begins to clinically improve, but oral doxycycline or azithromycin should be continued to complete a 14-day course [69, 70]. If the patient has a tubo-ovarian abscess, clindamycin or metronidazole should be used instead of doxycycline [70]. Complications of PID in pregnancy are fetal demise and preterm delivery, and long-term complications include infertility, ectopic pregnancy, and chronic pelvic pain [69].

Summary

Abdominal pain during pregnancy has both obstetric and non-obstetric causes. Up to 1% of pregnant women require an operation for a non-obstetric cause during their pregnancy, with appendicitis being the most common culprit. Though diagnosis can be challenging in pregnancy, assessment of abdominal pain during pregnancy should include evaluation of potential gynecologic, genitourinary, and gastrointestinal causes.

Key Points

- Abdominal pain in pregnancy is not always obstetric in origin.
- Abdominal pain in pregnancy can be diagnostically challenging due to anatomic and physiologic changes that occur during pregnancy.
- Ultrasound is the most common diagnostic tool to evaluate pelvic and abdominal pain during pregnancy and is safe to use.
- Appendicitis is the most common cause of non-obstetric emergency surgery in pregnancy, and diagnostic delay can lead to increased fetal mortality.
- Pregnancy and the use of assisted reproductive technology treatments increase the risk of ovarian torsion. Delay in diagnosis and surgical intervention can lead to increased fetal mortality and maternal morbidity.
- Physiologic changes in pregnancy promote ascending urinary tract infections, which without proper treatment can lead to premature delivery and low birth weight infants.

References

1. Diegelmann L. Nonobstetric Abdominal pain and surgical emergencies in pregnancy. Emerg Med Clin North Am. 2012;30(4):885–901.
2. Barber-Millet S, Bueno Lledó J, Granero Castro P, Gómez Gavara I, Ballester Pla N, García DR. Actualización en el manejo del abdomen agudo no obstétrico en la paciente gestante. Cir Esp. 2016;94(5):257–65.
3. Jones D, Wilson J, Warnock NG, Alexander DJ. Abdominal pain in pregnancy. BMJ. 2012;345:e6818.
4. Abbasi N, Patenaude V, Abenhaim HA. Management and outcomes of acute appendicitis in pregnancy—population-based study of over 7000 cases. BJOG. 2014;121(12):1509–14.
5. Longo SA, Moore RC, Canzoneri BJ, Robichaux A. Gastrointestinal conditions during pregnancy. Clin Colon Rectal Surg. 2010;23(2):80–9.
6. Erkek A, Anik Ilhan G, Yildizhan B, Aktan AO. Location of the appendix at the third trimester of pregnancy: a new approach to old dilemma. J Obstet Gynaecol. 2015;35(7):688–90.
7. Franca Neto AH, Amorim MM, Nobrega BM. Acute Appendicitis in pregnancy: literature review. Rev Assoc Med Bras. 2015;61(2):170–7.

8. Fonesca AL, Schuster KM, Kaplan LJ, Maung AA, Lui FY, Davis KA. The use of magnetic resonance imaging in the diagnosis of suspected appendicitis in pregnancy: shortened length of stay without increase in hospital charges. JAMA Surg. 2014;149(7):687–93.

9. Thompson MM, Kudla A, Chisholm CB. Appendicitis during pregnancy with a normal MRI. West J Emerg Med. 2014;15(6):652–4.

10. Drake FT, Kotagal M, Simmons LE, Parr Z, Dighe MK, Flum DR. Single institution and state-wide performance of ultrasound in diagnosing appendicitis in pregnancy. J Matern Fetal Neonatal Med. 2015;28(6):727–33.

11. Theilen LH, Mellnick VM, Longman RE, Tuuli MG, Odibo AO, Macones GA, Cahill AG. Utility of magnetic resonance imaging for suspected appendicitis in pregnant women. Am J Obstet Gynecol. 2015;212(3):345.e1–6.

12. Ramalingam V, LeBedis C, Kelly JR, Uyeda J, Soto JA, Anderson SW. Evaluation of a sequential multi-modality imaging algorithm for the diagnosis of acute appendicitis in the pregnant female. Emerg Radiol. 2015;22(2):125–32.

13. Bouyou J, Gaujoux S, Marcellin L, Leconte M, Goffinet F, Chapron C, Dousset B. Abdominal emergencies during pregnancy. J Visc Surg. 2015;152(6 Suppl):S105–15.

14. Aggenbach L, Zeeman GG, Cantineau AE, Gordijn SJ, Hofker HS. Impact of appendicitis during pregnancy: no delay in accurate diagnosis and treatment. Int J Surg. 2015;15:84–9.

15. Dalsgaard Jensen T, Penninga L. Appendicitis during pregnancy in a Greenlandic Inuit woman; antibiotic treatment as a bridge-to-surgery in a remote area. BMJ Case Rep. 2016;18:2016. doi:10.1136/bcr-2016-214722.

16. Knab LM, Boller AM, Mahvi DM. Cholecystitis. Surg Clin North Am. 2014;94(2):455–70.

17. de Bari O, Wang TY, Liu M, Paik CN, Portincasa P, Wang DQ. Cholesterol cholelithiasis in pregnant women: pathogenesis, prevention and treatment. Ann Hepatol. 2014;13(6):728–45.

18. Wu W, Faigel DO, Sun G, Yang Y. Non-radiation endoscopic retrograde cholangiopancreatography in the management of choledocholithiasis during pregnancy. Dig Endosc. 2014;26(6):691–700.

19. Jorge AM, Keswani RN, Veerappan A, Soper NJ, Gawron AJ. Non-operative management of symptomatic cholelithiasis in pregnancy is associated with frequent hospitalizations. J Gastrointest Surg. 2015;19(4):598–603.

20. Ibitoye BO, Adisa AO, Makinde ON, Ijarotimi AO. Prevalence and complications of gallstone disease among pregnant women in a Nigerian hospital. Int J Gynaecol Obstet. 2014;125(1):41–3.

21. Sun Y, Fan C, Wang S. Clinical analysis of 16 patients with acute pancreatitis in the third trimester of pregnancy. Int J Clin Exp Pathol. 2013;6(8):1696–701.

22. Gilbert A, Patenaude V, Abenhaim HA. Acute pancreatitis in pregnancy: a comparison of associated conditions, treatments and complications. J Perinat Med. 2014;42(5):565–70.

23. Kim JY, Jung SH, Choi HW, Song DJ, Jeong CY, Lee DH, Whang IS. Acute idiopathic pancreatitis in pregnancy: a case study. World J Gastroenterol. 2014;20(43):16364–7.

24. Cain MA, Ellis J, Vengrove MA, Wilcox B, Yankowitz J, Smulian JC. Gallstone and severe hypertriglyceride-induced pancreatitis in pregnancy. Obstet Gynecol Surv. 2015;70(9):577–83.

25. Abdullah B, Kathiresan Pillai T, Cheen LH, Ryan RJ. Severe acute pancreatitis in pregnancy. Case Rep Obstet Gynecol. 2015;2015:239068. doi:10.1155/2015/239068. Epub 2015 Jan 5

26. Xu Q, Wang S, Zhang Z. A 23-year, single-center, retrospective analysis of 36 cases of acute pancreatitis in pregnancy. Int J Gynaecol Obstet. 2015;130:123–6.

27. Hacker FM, Whalen PS, Lee VR, Caughey AB. Maternal and fetal outcomes of pancreatitis in pregnancy. Am J Obstet Gynecol. 2015;213(4):568.e1–5.

28. Bodner J, Windisch J, Bale R, Wetscher G, Mark W. Perforated right colonic diverticulitis complicating pregnancy at 37 weeks' gestation. Int J Colorectal Dis. 2005;20(4):381–2.

29. Pandeva I, Kumar S, Alvi A, Nosib H. Meckel's diverticulitis as a cause of an acute abdomen in the second trimester of pregnancy: laparoscopic management. Case Rep Obstet Gynecol. 2015;2015:835609. doi:10.1155/2015/835609. Epub 2015 Jan 11

30. Ribeiro Nascimento EF, Chechter M, Fonte FP, Puls N, Valenciano JS, Fernandes Filho CL, Nonose R, Bonassa CE, Martinez CA. Volvulus of the sigmoid colon during pregnancy: a case report. Case Rep Obstet Gynecol. 2012;2012:641093. doi:10.1155/2012/641093. Epub 2012 Feb 9
31. Palmucci S, Lanza ML, Gulino F, Scilletta B, Ettore GC. Diagnosis of a sigmoid volvulus in pregnancy: ultrasonography and magnetic resonance imaging findings. J Radiol Case Rep. 2014;8(2):54–62.
32. Atamanalp SS, Kisaoglu A, Ozogul B, Kantarci M, Disci E, Bulut OH, Aksungur N, Atamanalp RS. Sigmoid volvulus complicating pregnancy: a case report. Eur J Med. 2015;47(1):75–6.
33. Al Maksoud AM, Barsoum AK, Moneer MM. Sigmoid volvulus during pregnancy: a rare non-obstetric complication. Report of a case and review of the literature. Int J Surg Case Rep. 2015;17:61–4.
34. Ahmad A, Shing KK, Tan KK, Krasu M, Bickle I, Chong VH. Sigmoid volvulus in pregnancy: early diagnosis and intervention are important. Am J Emerg Med. 2014;32(5):491.e1–2.
35. Aftab Z, Toro A, Abdelaal A, Dasovky M, Gehani S, Abdel Mola A, Di Carlo I. Endoscopic reduction of a volvulus of the sigmoid colon in pregnancy: case report and a comprehensive review of the literature. World J Emerg Surg. 2014;9:41.
36. Hatch Q, Champagne BJ, Maykel JA, Davis BR, Johnson EK, Bleier JI, Francone TD, Steele SR. The impact of pregnancy on surgical Crohn disease: an analysis of the nationwide inpatient sample. J Surg Res. 2014;190(1):41–6.
37. van der Woude CJ, Metselaar HJ, Danese S. Management of gastrointestinal and liver diseases during pregnancy. Gut. 2014;63(6):1014–23.
38. Uma M. Pregnancy concerns in women with inflammatory bowel disease. Gastroenterol Hepatol. 2015;11(4):273–5.
39. McConnell RA, Mahadevan U. Pregnancy and the patient with inflammatory bowel disease: fertility, treatment, delivery and complications. Gastroenterol Clin North Am. 2016;45(2):285–301.
40. Mahadevan U, Matro R. Care of the pregnant patient with inflammatory bowel disease. Obstet Gynecol. 2015;126(2):401–12.
41. Nguyen GC, Seow CH, Maxwell C, Huang V, Leung Y, Jones J, Leontiadis GI, Tse F, Mahadevan U, van der Woude CJ, IBD in Pregnancy Consensus Group. The Toronto consensus statements for the management of inflammatory bowel disease in pregnancy. Gastroenterology. 2016;150(3):734–57.e1.
42. Bar-Gil Shitrit A, Grisaru-Granovsky S, Ben Ya'acov A, Goldin E. Management of inflammatory bowel disease during pregnancy. Dig Dis Sci. 2016. [Epub ahead of print].
43. Zielinski R, Searing K, Deibel M. Gastrointestinal distress in pregnancy: prevalence, assessment, and treatment of 5 common minor discomforts. J Perinat Neonatal Nurs. 2015;29(1):23–31.
44. Body C, Christie JA. Gastrointestinal diseases in pregnancy: nausea, vomiting, hyperemesis gravidarum, gastroesophageal reflux disease, constipation, and diarrhea. Gastroenterol Clin North Am. 2016;45(2):267–83.
45. Goel B, Rani J, Huria A, Gupta P, Dalal U. Perforated duodenal ulcer—a rare cause of acute abdomen in pregnancy. J Clin Diagn Res. 2014;8(9):OD03–4.
46. Erez O, Maymon E, Mazor M. Acute gastric ulcer perforation in a 35 weeks' nulliparous patient with gastric banding. Am J Obstet Gynecol. 2004;191(5):1721–2.
47. Johnson P, Mount K, Graziano S. Functional bowel disorders in pregnancy: effect on quality of life, evaluation and management. Acta Obstet Gynecol Scand. 2014;93(9):874–9.
48. Griffin C. Probiotics in obstetrics and gynaecology. Aust N Z J Obstet Gynaecol. 2015;55(3):201–9.
49. Rungsiprakarn P, Laopaiboon M, Sangkomkamhang US, Lumbiganon P, Pratt JJ. Interventions for treating constipation in pregnancy. Cochrane Database Syst Rev. 2015;9:CD011448. doi:10.1002/14651858.CD011448.pub2.

50. Tsai H, Kuo T, Chung M, Lin M, Kang C, Tsai Y. Acute abdomen in early pregnancy due to ovarian torsion following successful in vitro fertilization treatment. Taiwan J Obstet Gynecol. 2015;54:438–41.
51. Chang S, Yen C, Lo L, Lee C, Liang C. Surgical intervention for maternal ovarian torsion in pregnancy. Taiwan J Obstet Gynecol. 2011;50:458–62.
52. Zucchini S, Marra E. Diagnosis of emergencies/urgencies in gynecology and during the first trimester of pregnancy. J Ultrasound. 2014;17:41–6.
53. Sun Y, Liu L, Di J. Isolated tubal torsion in the third trimester of pregnancy: a case report and review of the literature. J Res Med Sci. 2014;19(11):1106–9.
54. Bhavsar AK, Gelner EJ, Shorma T. Common questions about the evaluation of acute pelvic pain. Am Fam Physician. 2016;93(1):41–8.
55. Minig L, Otaño L, Cruz P, Patrono MG, Botazzi C, Zapardiel I. Laparoscopic surgery for treating adnexal masses during the first trimester of pregnancy. J Min Access Surg. 2016;12(1):22–5.
56. Haan J, Verheecke M, Amant F. Management of ovarian cysts and cancer in pregnancy. Facts Views Vis Obgyn. 2015;7(1):25–31.
57. Huancahuari N. Emergences in early pregnancy. Emerg Med Clin N Am. 2012;30:837–47.
58. Radhika B, Naik K, Shreelatha S, Vana H. Case series: pregnancy outcome in patients with uterine fibroids. J Clin Diagn Res. 2015;9(10):QR01–4.
59. Currie A, Bradley E, McEwen M, Al-Shabibi N, Willson P. Laparoscopic approach to fibroid torsion presenting as an acute abdomen in pregnancy. J Soc Laparoendosc Surg. 2013;17:665–7.
60. Lee HJ, Norwitz ER, Shaw J. Contemporary management of fibroids in pregnancy. Rev Obstet Gynecol. 2010;3(1):20–7.
61. Zaima A, Ash A. Fibroid in pregnancy: characteristics, complications, and management. Postgrad Med J. 2011;87:819–28. doi:10.1136/postgradmedj-2011-130319.
62. Guinto V, Guia B, Festin M, Dowswell T. Different antibiotic regiments for treating asymptomatic bacteriuria in pregnancy. Cochrana Database Syst Rev 2010;(9).
63. Matuszkiewicz-Rowinska J, Malyszko J, Wieliczko M. URinary tract infections in pregnancy: old and new unresolved diagnostic and therapeutic problems. Arch Med Sci. 2015;11(1):67–77.
64. Delzell J, Lefevre M. Urinary tract infections during pregnancy. Am Fam Physician. 2000;61(3):713–20.
65. Artero A, Alberola J, Eiros J, Nogueira J, Cano A. Pyelonephritis in pregnancy. How adequate is empirical treatment? Rev Esp Quimioter. 2013;26(1):30–3.
66. Nash Z, Mascarenhas L. Renal calculi in pregnancy? The role of ultralow-dose CT. BMJ Case Rep. 2013. doi:10.1136/bcr-2013-009021.
67. Adanur S, Ziypak T, Bedir F, Yapanoglu T, Aydin H, Yilmaz M, et al. Ureteroscopy and holmium laser lithotripsy: Is this procedure safe in pregnant women with ureteral stones at different locations? Archivio Italiano di Urologia e Andrologia. 2014;2:86–9.
68. Stothers L, Lee LM. Renal colic in pregnancy. J Urol. 1992;148(5):1383–7.
69. Ford GW, Decker CF. Pelvic inflammatory disease. Disease-a-Month. 2016.
70. Sweet R. Treatment of acute pelvic inflammatory disease. Infect Dis Obstret Gynecol. 2011;1-10.
71. Blanchard AC, Pastorek JG, Weeks T. Pelvic inflammatory disease during pregnancy. South Med J. 1987;80(11):1363–5.
72. Yip L, Sweeny P, Bock B. Acute suppurative salpingitis with concomitant intrauterine pregnancy. Am J Emerg Med. 1993;11:476–9.

Chapter 13
Imaging Considerations in Pregnancy

Diana Ladkany and Kerri Layman

Introduction

Women account for 50.8% of the population, and in 2011, 60/1000 women of child-bearing age (15–44) were pregnant [1]. Pregnant women often present to the emergency department (ED) for both pregnancy- and nonpregnancy-related medical emergencies. ED management often involves the difficult decision of how to use medical diagnostic imaging appropriately and safely without placing the mother and the fetus at unnecessary risk. Multiple factors play a role in deciding how and when to using imaging to aid in diagnosis; therefore, understanding the risks and benefits of each imaging modality is essential. Imaging studies commonly used in the ED include ultrasonography, X-ray, computed tomography (CT) scan, magnetic resonance imaging (MRI), and nuclear medicine. Ultrasound is used most often for assessing the fetus and has been found to be safe in all studies to date, but has its limitations. The most controversial modes of imaging are those that use ionizing radiation such as X-ray and CT. MRI is considered safe in pregnancy, but can be time-consuming and is not readily available in all departments. The emergency physician must possess the appropriate body of knowledge to counsel their pregnant patients on the best imaging modality for diagnosis of their condition. Importantly, a necessary diagnostic test should not be withheld from a pregnant patient out of concern for the possible risk to the fetus.

D. Ladkany, B.S., M.D. (✉)
Department of Emergency Medicine, MedStar Washington Hospital Center and MedStar
Georgetown University, 110 Irving St. NW, Washington, DC 20010, USA
e-mail: ladkanyd@gmail.com

K. Layman, B.S.F.S., M.D., R.D.M.S.
Department of Emergency Medicine, MedStar Georgetown University Hospital and MedStar
Washington Hospital Center, 3800 Reservoir Road NW, Washington, DC 20007, USA
e-mail: kllayman2000@yahoo.com

© Springer International Publishing AG 2017
J. Borhart (ed.), *Emergency Department Management of Obstetric Complications*,
DOI 10.1007/978-3-319-54410-6_13

Ultrasound

The most common method of imaging used during pregnancy is ultrasound. Ultrasound is universally accepted as safe during pregnancy. Ultrasound uses high-frequency sound waves to produce images. The sound waves emit heat, leading to a theoretical risk of thermal damage when the acoustic output is too high. Higher acoustic output is necessary when using Doppler imaging to determine blood flow; thus, the use of Doppler should be limited during pregnancy. Despite the theoretical risk, there have been no studies documenting adverse fetal effects from diagnostic ultrasound, including the use of Doppler imaging [2].

The primary benefits of ultrasound are its portability and ability to provide real-time bedside imaging. For this reason, along with its safety profile, ultrasound is the primary imaging modality of choice for fetal imaging. Measurements including fetus size and fetal heart rate are obtained quickly and safely. Ultrasound is not only useful for evaluating the fetus but can be very helpful in diagnosing certain emergent conditions in the mother as well such as appendicitis, cholecystitis, and ovarian pathology.

Ultrasound has the benefit of evaluating structures functionally, anatomically, and dynamically as the patient's condition evolves. In addition to static imaging, the ability to utilize Doppler imaging allows proper evaluation of blood flow in structures of concern. This is particularly pertinent when evaluating a patient with concern for ovarian torsion. While ultrasound of the ovaries is the modality of choice in the first and early second trimester, full visualization of the adnexa can become challenging in the late second and third trimesters.

Despite its many advantages, ultrasound has significant limitations. These limitations include maternal obesity, operator skill, and image quality [3]. When evaluating the abdomen of a gravid woman, the uterus and fetus may obstruct the ultrasound images of the organ of interest, especially later in pregnancy. Furthermore, ultrasound is not ideal for hollow viscous imaging such as the intestines, pancreatic imaging, bone, and neurologic imaging. Chapter 2 "Emergency Department Ultrasound in Pregnancy" provides a detailed discussion on the use of point-of-care ultrasound for the ED evaluation of the pregnant patient.

Ionizing Radiation Including X-Rays and CT

Ionizing radiation during pregnancy may expose the fetus; however, this has been found to be limited. The estimated radiation dose a fetus receives is dependent on the type of study being acquired, proximity of the uterus to the anatomic location of the scan plane, patient size, X-ray technique, and whether or not protective mechanisms are used such as lead covering of the abdomen and pelvis.

The clinical effect of radiation on a fetus depends on the age of gestation and the amount of radiation. The most vulnerable period is 8–15 weeks of gestation [4].

Above levels of 100–200 mGy, there is a risk of teratogenesis and pregnancy loss; however, medical diagnostic testing uses radiation doses far below this threshold. In the very early stages of pregnancy (<4 weeks), the embryo is somewhat protected from possible teratogenic exposure due to the totipotent or pluripotent nature of the cells, which allows the abnormal cells to be replaced by nearby cells [5]. The effect of teratogenic exposure before 4 weeks tends to be "all or none," meaning the exposure results in the death of the embryo or no consequence. Between 4 and 8 weeks, the embryo is at a higher risk of congenital anomalies of the organs, skeleton, or genitals [3]. Between weeks 8–15 when organogenesis occurs, exposure to radiation levels of greater than 100 mGy may cause fetal demise, intellectual deficit, or microcephaly (Table 13.1. Effects of gestational age).

Ionizing radiation has also been linked to an increased risk of malignancy. The data used to make this link has been extrapolated from the cancer rates following atomic bomb exposure in Hiroshima and Nagasaki, as well as the aftereffects of the Chernobyl disaster. Cumulative exposure to 100 mGy of ionizing radiation is associated with increased risk of developing malignancy; below this level, cancer cannot be correlated with radiation exposure. Diagnostic medical tests involving ionizing radiation utilize significantly less radiation than 100 mGy.

The American College of Obstetricians and Gynecologists (ACOG) supports the use of medical diagnostic imaging when the radiation exposure is less than 50 mGy, as fetal anomalies have not been reported below this level [2]. However, the use of ionizing radiation studies should not be withheld in a pregnant patient regardless of the radiation dose if there is an emergent clinical indication. Appropriate and timely diagnosis and treatment of the emergency affecting the mother is the safest way to protect the fetus.

Table 13.1 Effects of gestational age and radiation dose on radiation-induced teratogenesis

Gestational period	Effects	Estimated threshold dose[a]
Before implantation (0–2 weeks after conception)	Death of embryo or no consequence (all or none)	50–100 mGy
Organogenesis (2–8 weeks after conception)	Congenital anomalies (skeleton, eyes, genitals)	200 mGy
	Growth retardation	200–250 mGy
Fetal period		
8–15 Weeks	Severe mental retardation (high risk)[b]	60–310 mGy
	Intellectual deficit	25 IQ point loss per gray
	Microcephaly	200 mGy
16–25 Weeks	Severe mental retardation (low risk)	250–280 mGy

[a]Data based on results of animal studies, epidemiologic studies of survivors of the atomic bombings in Japan, and studies of groups exposed to radiation for medical reasons (e.g. radiation therapy for carcinoma of the uterus)
[b]Because this is a period of rapid neuronal development and migration
Patel SJ, Reede DL, Katz DS, et al. Imaging the pregnant patient for nonobstetric conditions: Algorithms and radiation dose considerations. RadioGraphics 2007;27:1705–1722. With permission

X-ray is the most common form of ionizing radiation used during pregnancy. Most X-rays are very low-dose examinations (<0.1 mGy) and therefore pose almost no risk to the fetus. Very low-dose X-rays include the cervical spine, chest (two views), and any extremity films. Low- to moderate-dose examinations (0–10 mGy) include abdominal, thoracic, and lumbar spine X-rays (Table 13.2. Fetal radiation doses).

The highest doses of ionizing radiation are from CT scans. For example, a CT angiography of the chest to rule out pulmonary embolism exposes the mother to anywhere between 13 and 40 mGy of radiation with the average being about 15 mGy depending on the radiology protocol and type of machinery [6]. The fetal exposure is much less, between 0.01 and 0.66 mGy. A CT of the abdomen and pelvis during pregnancy exposes a fetus to approximately 25 mGy. CT of the head, neck, and extremities usually results in only negligible scatter radiation to the fetus [6].

Table 13.2 Fetal radiation doses associated with common radiological axaminations [6, 21, 22]

Type of examination	Fetal absorbed dose[a] (mGy)
Very low-dose examinations (<0.1 mGy)	
• Cervical spine X-ray (AP and lateral)	<0.001
• Any extremity X-ray	<0.001
• Chest X-ray (two views)	0.0005–0.01
Low- to moderate-dose examinations (0–10 mGy)	
Radiography	
• Thoracic spine X-ray	0.003
• Abdominal X-ray	0.1–3
• Lumbar spine X-ray	1–10
• Intravenous pyelography	5–10
• Double-contrast barium enema	1–20
CT	
• Head, neck, or extremity[b]	0–10
• Chest CT or CT pulmonary angiography	0.01–0.66
Nuclear medicine	
• Low-dose perfusion scintigraphy	0.1–0.5
• V/Q scintigraphy	0.1–0.8
Higher-dose examinations (10–50 mGy)	
• Abdominal CT	1.3–35
• Pelvic CT	10–50
• Abdomen and pelvis	13–25
• Aortic angiography of chest, abdomen, pelvis with or without contrast agent	6.7–56
• Coronary artery angiography	0.1–3
• Nonenhanced CT of abdomen and pelvis to evaluate for nephrolithiasis	10–11

CT computed tomography, *V/Q* ventilation/perfusion
[a]Fetal dose varies with gestational age, maternal body habitus, and exact acquisition parameters
[b]Most authors report fetal dose from the head, neck, or extremity CT close to zero (negligible scatter)

In the event that imaging with CT is necessary to diagnose an emergent medical condition in a pregnant patient, the risks and benefits should be discussed while trying to highlight the importance of diagnosis over radiation, since the fetal exposure is quite limited [7]. It is considered appropriate to use CT scanning in pregnancy if the risk of non-diagnosis or worsening of disease outweighs the risk of radiation exposure. Despite its generally accepted safety, radiation doses should be kept As Low As Reasonably Achievable, commonly known as the ALARA principle.

Iodinated intravenous (IV) contrast agents such as iohexol are frequently utilized to enhance CT imaging, but do not go without risk. In all patients there is the possibility of mild adverse effects, such as flushing and pain at injection site, as well as serious effects such as anaphylactoid reactions and acute kidney injury (due to cytotoxic effects of contrast on the tubules as well as renal vasoconstriction). In pregnant women, IV iohexol crosses the placental barrier. Since it is excreted through the urinary system, iohexol stays within the amniotic fluid, is not fully cleared, and can be found in fetal tissue [8]. In one case report, iodinated contrast material was found in the fetal intestines after birth but was cleared after infant stooling increased. No harm to the infants was found [9]. Although no reports of fetal hypothyroidism and teratogenic effects from IV iodinated contrast have been found, it is best to avoid contrast when at all possible to follow the ALARA principle. If contrast is necessary to make an accurate diagnosis, as is the case in pulmonary embolus and trauma evaluation, it is reasonable to use. Iohexol and most iodinated contrast have been categorized as Food and Drug Administration (FDA) pregnancy class B drugs. A very small amount of iohexol (less than 1%) is excreted into breast milk, but there is no need to for lactating women who receive IV contrast to interrupt breastfeeding [8]. Oral contrast agents are not absorbed by the patient and do not cause harm in pregnancy.

Magnetic Resonance Imaging

Magnetic resonance imaging (MRI) uses a powerful magnetic field and radio waves to produce an image based on the energy released from protons within the body [10]. This form of imaging does not use any ionizing radiation, and therefore the risks during pregnancy are minimal. The major theoretical risk of MRI during pregnancy is in the first trimester during which organogenesis is occurring. Experts postulate the possibility of acoustic damage to developing neural systems and the possibility for tissue overheating, but these risks are purely theoretical and lack practical evidence. There has been no evidence of harm with the use of MRI during pregnancy. In addition to ultrasound, emergency clinicians should feel comfortable using MRI as a first-line imaging choice, even in the first trimester of pregnancy. MRI should be considered instead of CT imaging whenever the clinical scenario allows [11]. A major limiting factor for using MRI in the emergency department is that it takes much longer than CT to acquire images. Therefore in an unstable patient, CT may be preferred over MRI to make a timely diagnosis.

Gadolinium-based contrast is often used to enhance MRI images. However, gadolinium is a class C pregnancy drug due to its potential toxic effects. The chelated form of gadolinium is not harmful; however, the free form is highly toxic [12]. Gadolinium crosses the placenta and is not cleared effectively from fetal circulation, which can result in possible carcinogenesis and growth retardation, as seen in animal studies [4]. No prospective studies have been conducted in pregnant women, due to the demonstrated toxic animal studies. Given the risk, gadolinium should be avoided in pregnant patients. Lactating women who receive gadolinium do not have to interrupt breastfeeding.

Nuclear Medicine and Fluoroscopy

Nuclear medicine studies use radioisotopes to "tag" a chemical agent and produce an image showing the physiologic function or dysfunction of an organ. Nuclear medicine studies are employed frequently in the ED to evaluate for coronary artery disease (nuclear stress test) and pulmonary emboli (ventilation/perfusion or V/Q lung scanning). Technetium 99 m is the isotope commonly used in these scans and is considered safe in pregnancy. However, radioactive iodine (iodine 131), an isotope often used in thyroid imaging, readily crosses the placenta and should be avoided in pregnant patients as there is a theoretical risk to the developing thyroid gland and may cause fetal hypothyroidism. Nuclear scans do expose the mother and fetus to some ionizing radiation, generally less than 5 mGy in the case of V/Q scans [2]. Additionally, radionuclide compounds are excreted in breast milk.

Finally, interventional radiology is often utilized to help with procedures that may be technically challenging or high risk such as lumbar puncture, central line or medi-port placements, biopsies, and embolization of bleeding vessels. Many of these procedures employ ionizing radiation (fluoroscopy), but some can be done under ultrasound. When possible, it is best to avoid fluoroscopy since it requires multiple X-rays in succession.

Common Diagnostic Scenarios and Suggested Imaging Strategies

Trauma

Trauma is the leading cause of maternal death from non-obstetric causes during pregnancy, and one in every 12 pregnancies is affected by some form of trauma [14]. Ultrasound is often utilized in the emergency department evaluation of trauma. A focused assessment with sonography for trauma (FAST) exam can be done to evaluate for free fluid within the abdomen. Although some small amount of free pelvic fluid can be expected in pregnancy, it is likely going to be very minimal and is usually associated with ovarian hyperstimulation or ovarian cysts. In a trauma setting, greater than 2 mm of free fluid in the pelvis is unlikely to be physiologic [13].

Another valuable use of ultrasound in the trauma evaluation is to quickly evaluate the fetus. This can provide information on gestational age of the fetus and its viability (generally >23 weeks), fetal heartbeat, and some general information about the placenta such as the location. Ultrasound is insensitive to diagnose placental abruption [14].

In cases of significant trauma, physicians should not hesitate to utilize CT despite the radiation dose to the fetus. Evaluating the possible injuries in trauma quickly is essential; therefore, using MRI is usually not preferred.

Pulmonary Embolism

The optimal imaging approach to diagnose pulmonary embolism (PE) in pregnancy has been extensively debated. Ventilation/perfusion (V/Q) scan exposes the fetus to 0.1–0.8 mGy of radiation; CT angiography scan of the chest exposes the fetus to 0.01–0.66 mGy of radiation. The exact exposure depends on the gestational age of the fetus with the third trimester having the highest exposure levels to the fetus [15]. Both imaging modalities confer radiation doses well below the threshold associated with fetal harm. However, risks to the mother must also be considered, and CT angiography confers higher maternal radiation exposure compared to V/Q scan, particularly to breast tissue. CT has the benefit of identifying alternate pathology; V/Q scans are occasionally indeterminate necessitating additional imaging studies. It is the author's opinion that both CT angiography and V/Q scans are equally justifiable for the pregnant patient. The authors prefer CT angiography.

Appendicitis

Appendicitis affects approximately one in every 1500 pregnancies and is more common in the second trimester [16]. A sequential imaging approach may be necessary to diagnose acute appendicitis, beginning with ultrasound. However, due to the size of the gravid uterus, the utility of ultrasound may be limited, particularly in the late stage of pregnancy. The nonvisualization rates of ultrasound can be as high as 90% and are dependent on maternal factors, term of pregnancy, and operator skill [3]. If ultrasound is nondiagnostic, MRI is the imaging modality of choice to evaluate the appendix [12]. If MRI is unavailable, CT scan may be performed in consultation with an obstetrician and the patient as abdominal/pelvic CT is a higher-dose examination (10–50 mGy fetal dose).

Kidney Stone

Nephrolithiasis can affect one in every 200–2500 pregnancies. In the case of renal colic, ultrasound is diagnostic 60% of the time, but if it is inconclusive, MR urography may be considered [12]. If MR urography is unavailable, non-contrast CT may be necessary, again in consultation with the patient and their obstetrician.

Gallbladder Disease

Diagnosing hepatobiliary pathology is also a challenge during pregnancy. Due to higher progesterone levels in pregnancy, which slows gallbladder emptying, 1–3% of pregnant women will have biliary stones, and up to 30% will have biliary sludge seen on ultrasound. Fortunately, acute cholecystitis affects less than 1% of pregnant women [16]. The best method of diagnosing acute cholecystitis is ultrasound; however, MRI or CT may be necessary in the later stages of pregnancy. In some cases, if cholecystitis has been diagnosed, percutaneous cholecystostomy tube placement by interventional radiology may be used until cholecystectomy can be more safely done after delivery of the fetus [17].

Stroke and Intracranial Hemorrhage

MRI is the superior imaging modality when evaluating the neurologic system. Due to the thromboembolic state of pregnancy, pregnant women are at higher risk for cerebral vascular accidents. Approximately 11–26 out of 100,000 pregnant or immediately postpartum women will have a stroke [18]. Non-contrast head CT scan is appropriate in pregnant women to evaluate for intracerebral hemorrhage. MRI is the preferred method of imaging to evaluate for ischemic stroke [19]. Since gadolinium should be avoided in pregnancy, CT with iodinated contrast can be used if necessary to fully image cerebral vasculature, which may help guide therapy [20].

Summary

The emergency physician will often be faced with deciding which mode of imaging is appropriate and necessary for a pregnant patient. Many factors affect this decision including the stage of pregnancy, the urgency of the diagnosis, and what specifically is being evaluated. Ultrasound and MRI are the safest imaging modalities to evaluate the mother and the fetus and are not associated with risk to the pregnancy; however, gadolinium contrast should be avoided. In many cases ionizing radiation such as CT is necessary to make an accurate and timely diagnosis, especially in the acute setting of trauma. Necessary diagnostic tests should not be withheld from a pregnant patient out of concern for possible risk to the fetus.

Key Points

- Ultrasound is the preferred initial mode of imaging for most diagnoses when feasible and appropriate, especially in fetal and pelvic imaging.
- CT imaging with IV iodinated contrast is safe and should be used first in certain situations, most notably in trauma.
- MRI is preferred over CT for most diagnostic purposes during pregnancy; however, IV gadolinium contrast should be avoided.
- Ionizing radiation poses a risk of teratogenicity at >100 mGy of radiation, and radiation exposure should be limited during pregnancy. However, medical imaging uses lower doses of radiation, and therefore fetal exposure is usually significantly lower than this threshold and should be used when necessary.
- In an emergency, the emergency physician should use any imaging necessary to make an accurate and timely diagnosis to ensure the best outcome for both the mother and the fetus.

References

1. Census Bureau. Measuring childbearing patterns in the United States. 2011. www.census.gov. July 2016.
2. Gynecologists, The American College of Obstetricians and. Committee Opinion No. 656: guidelines for diagnostic imaging during pregnancy and lactation. Committee Opin. 2016.
3. Baysinger CL. Imaging during pregnancy. Anesth Analg. 2010.
4. Gomes M, Matias A, Macedo F. Risks to the fetus from diagnostic imaging during pregnancy: review and proposal of a clinical protocol. Pediatr Radiol. 2015:45:1916–29.
5. Goodman TR, Amurao M. Medical imaging radiation safety for the female patient: rationale and implementation. Radiographics. 2012;32:1829–37.
6. McCollough CH, Schueler BA, Atwell TD, et al. Radiation exposure in pregnancy: when should we be concerned? Radiographics. 2007;27:909–17.
7. Hendee WR, O'Connor MK. Radiation risks of medical imaging: separating fact from fantasy. Radiology. 2012;264(2):312–21.
8. Beckett KR, Moriarity AK, Langer JM. Safe use of contrast media: What the radiologist needs to know. Radiographics. 2015;35(6):1738–50.
9. Moon AJ, Katzberg RW, Sherman MP. Transplacental passage of iohexal. J Pediatr. 2000;136(4):548–9.
10. National Institute of Biomedical Imaging and Bioengineering: MRI. n.d. https://www.nibib.nih.gov/science-education/science-topics/magnetic-resonance-imaging-mri.
11. Masselli G, Derme M, Laghi F, et al. Evaluating the acute abdomen in the pregnant patient. Radiol Clin North Am. 2015;53(6):1309–25.

12. McGahan JP, Lamba R, Coakley FV. Imaging non-obstetrical causes of abdominal pain in the pregnant patient. Appl Radiol. 2010;39(11):10–25.
13. Hussain ZJ, Figueroa R, Budorick NE. How much free fluid can a pregnant patient have? Assessment of pelvic free fluid in pregnant patients without antecedent trauma. J Trauma. 2011;70(6):1420–3.
14. Jain V, Chari R, Maslovitz S, et al. Guidelines for the management of a pregnant trauma patient. J Obstet Gynaecol Can. 2015;37(6):553–74.
15. Niemann T, Nicolas G, Roser HW, et al. Imaging for suspected pulmonary embolism in pregnancy-what about the fetal dose? A comprehensive review of the literature. Insights Imaging. 2010;1(5-6):361–372.
16. Gilo NB, Amini D, Landy HJ. Appendicitis and cholecystitis in pregnancy. Clin Obstet Gynecol. 2009;52(4):586–96.
17. Akhan O, Akinci D, Ozmen MN. Percutaneous cholecystostomy. Eur J Radiol. 2002;43(3):229–36.
18. Davie CA, O'Brien P. Stroke and pregnancy. J Neurol Neurosurg Psychiatry. 2008;79(3):240–5.
19. Del Zotto E, Giossi A, Volonghi I, et al. Ischemic stroke during pregnancy and puerperium. Stroke Res Treat. 2011:606780.
20. Chen MM, Coakley FV, Kaimal A, et al. Guidelines for computed tomography and magnetic resonance imaging use during pregnancy and lactation. Obstet Gynecol. 2008;112(2 Pt 1):333–40.
21. Tirada N, Dreizin D, Khati NJ, et al. Imaging pregnant and lactating patients. Radiographics. 2015;55:691–696
22. Tremblay E, Therasse E, Thomassin-Naggara I, et al. Quality initiatives: guidelines for the use of medical imaging during pregnancy and lactation. Radiographics. 2012;32:897–911.

Index